SAFETY & ACCIDENT PREVENTION

This new series is designed to meet the growing demand for current, accessible information about the increasingly popular wellness approach to personal health. The result of a collaborative effort by a highly professional writing, editorial, and publishing team, the *Wellness* series consists of 16 volumes, each on a single topic. Each volume in this attractively produced series combines original material with carefully selected readings, relevant statistical data, and illustrations. The series objectives are to increase awareness of the value of a wellness approach to personal health and to help the reader become a more informed consumer of health-related information. Employing a critical thinking approach, each volume includes a variety of assessment tools, discusses basic concepts, suggests key questions, and provides the reader with a list of resources for further exploration.

James K. Jackson	Wellness: AIDS, STD, & Other Communicable Diseases
Richard G. Schlaadt	Wellness: Alcohol Use & Abuse
Richard G. Schlaadt	Wellness: Drugs, Society, & Behavior
Robert E. Kime	Wellness: Environment & Health
Gary Klug & Janice Lettunich	Wellness: Exercise & Physical Fitness
James D. Porterfield & Richard St. Pierre	Wellness: Healthful Aging
Robert E. Kime	Wellness: The Informed Health Consumer
Paula F. Ciesielski	Wellness: Major Chronic Diseases
Robert E. Kime	Wellness: Mental Health
Judith S. Hurley	Wellness: Nutrition & Health
Robert E. Kime	Wellness: Pregnancy, Childbirth, & Parenting
David C. Lawson	Wellness: Safety & Accident Prevention
Randall R. Cottrell	Wellness: Stress Management
Richard G. Schlaadt	Wellness: Tobacco & Health
Randall R. Cottrell	Wellness: Weight Control
Judith S. Hurley & Richard G. Schlaadt	Wellness: The Wellness Life-Style

SAFETY & ACCIDENT PREVENTION

David C. Lawson

WELLNESS

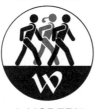

A MODERN
LIFE-STYLE
LIBRARY

The Dushkin Publishing Group, Inc./Sluice Dock, Guilford, CT 06437

Library of Congress Catalog Card Number: 91-061925
Manufactured in the United States of America
First Edition, First Printing
ISBN: 0-87967-864-X

Library of Congress Cataloging-in-Publication Data

Lawson, David C., Safety & Accident Prevention (Wellness)
    1. Accidents—Prevention. 2. Home accidents—Prevention. 3. Safety education. I. Title. II. Series.
HV675   613.69   91-061925   ISBN 0-87967-864-X

Please see page 145 for credits.

The procedures and explanations given in this publication are based on research and consultation with medical and nursing authorities. To the best of our knowledge, these procedures and explanations reflect currently accepted medical practice; nevertheless, they cannot be considered absolute and universal recommendations. For individual application, treatment suggestions must be considered in light of the individual's health, subject to a doctor's specific recommendations. The authors and the publisher disclaim responsibility for any adverse effects resulting directly or indirectly from the suggested procedures, from any undetected errors, or from the reader's misunderstanding of the text.

DAVID C. LAWSON

David C. Lawson received his doctorate in safety education from West Virginia University in 1969. He is a past president and former member of the board of directors of the American Driver Traffic Safety Education Association. He has also served on the board of governors of the American Association of Physical Health Education, Recreation, and Dance (AAPHERD), as chair of the Department of Health Education at Oregon State University, and as the chair of the Governors' Motorcycle Advisory Committee, a post to which he was appointed by the governor of the state of Oregon. Dr. Lawson is currently a fellow in the American Academy of Safety Education, associate professor and coordinator of the Occupational Health and Safety Program at Oregon State University, and the director of two federally and state-funded research projects.

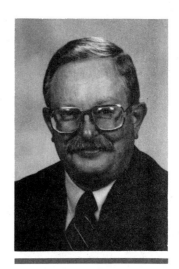

WELLNESS:
A Modern Life-Style Library

General Editors
Robert E. Kime, Ph.D.
Richard G. Schlaadt, Ed.D.

Authors
Paula F. Ciesielski, M.D.
Randall R. Cottrell, Ed.D.
Judith S. Hurley, M.S., R.D.
James K. Jackson, M.D.
Robert E. Kime, Ph.D.
Gary A. Klug, Ph.D.
David C. Lawson, Ph.D.
Janice Lettunich, M.S.
James D. Porterfield
Richard St. Pierre, Ph.D.
Richard G. Schlaadt, Ed.D.

Developmental Staff
Irving Rockwood, Program Manager
Paula Edelson, Series Editor
Maggie Hostetler, Developmental Editor
Wendy Connal, Administrative Assistant
Jason J. Marchi, Editorial Assistant

Editing Staff
John S. L. Holland, Managing Editor
Elizabeth Jewell, Copy Editor
Diane Barker, Editorial Assistant
Mary L. Strieff, Art Editor
Robert Reynolds, Illustrator

Production and Design Staff
Brenda S. Filley, Production Manager
Whit Vye, Cover Design and Logo
Jeremiah B. Lighter, Text Design
Libra Ann Cusack, Typesetting Supervisor
Charles Vitelli, Designer
Meredith Scheld, Graphics Assistant
Steve Shumaker, Graphics Assistant
Lara M. Johnson, Graphics Assistant
Juliana Arbo, Typesetter
Richard Tietjen, Editorial Systems Analyst

Preface

ACCIDENT PREVENTION IS a subject that rarely makes the 6-o'clock news or the front page of the newspaper. Unlike earthquakes, war, famine, and urban violence, preventing accidents is seldom considered newsworthy. But what most Americans don't realize is that for the first 36 years of our lives, we are more likely to lose our lives because of an accident than because of cancer or heart disease. Accidents, fatal or otherwise, are also costly as well. In 1989 the price tag for accidents ran just shy of $150 billion dollars. When we realize that most accidents are preventable, the toll they exact in lives lost, injuries sustained, and property damaged is astoundingly high.

In the following pages you will find more statistics that might make you think twice about the frequency with which accidents occur. Beyond the statistics, *Safety & Accident Prevention* examines different types of accidents—job-related, vehicular, household, recreational, and fire-related—almost all of which we as health consumers have the opportunity to prevent. Remember, it is estimated that 90 percent of accidents are due to human error. It is only through education, forethought, and preparation that we can secure an accident-free future for ourselves and those around us.

This is not a definitive work, but rather a place to begin. the central objective of this book is not to make you into an instant expert on safety and accident prevention but to help you learn to *think critically* about this important topic. Only then will you be able to distinguish safety myth from safety fact, and only then will you be an informed and safe health consumer.

David C. Lawson
Corvallis, OR

Contents

1

Accident Prevention
Page 1

2

Safety on the Road
Page 26

5

Fires and
Occupational
Safety
Page 94

FIGURES

1

Accident Prevention

now and then
there is a person born
who is so unlucky
that he runs into accidents
which started out to happen
to somebody else.

—Don Marquis, *archy says,* xli.

WHEN ANDY had his accident, he was an 18-year-old high school senior in a small town in the Midwest. An average student who excelled in basketball, he was planning to join the Air Force after graduation. Fast, daredevil driving was his claim to fame among his fellow students. One afternoon when his parents were away, Andy invited some friends over to watch a football game. During the course of the afternoon they drank some beers and decided to take a drive into the nearby big city. In the car with Andy were his girlfriend, Candace, and his friends, Kevin and Robert.

On the expressway Andy decided to open up and let his car fly, reaching speeds as high as 100 mph. Driving mostly in the left lane, Andy flashed his lights to signal slower drivers to move over. However, he failed to anticipate one circumstance—a car pulling a trailer in the left lane at 50 mph. He reported later that he saw it at the last minute, too late to slow down. To avoid a collision, he swerved onto the median and lost control of the car.

FIGURE 1.1

Accidental Death Rates by Age, 1989

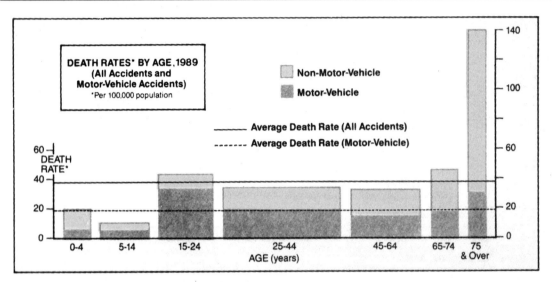

Source: National Safety Council, *Accident Facts,* 1990, p. 14.

The total number of accidental deaths among any given age group is determined by 2 factors—the size of the group and its rate of accidental death. The height of the bars in the above chart represents the death rate for each group. The width of the bars depicts its size (in proportion to the total population).

After hitting a guardrail, his car careened back across the highway lanes without hitting another vehicle, only to smash head-on into a tree. Andy was wearing a seat belt; his friends were not. Andy was uninjured, but Candace and Robert were killed instantly. Kevin was thrown from the car and suffered a severe head injury. A year and a half later he has regained a limited ability to talk and walk but will be an invalid for the rest of his life.

Elinor was a 76-year-old widow living by herself in California. She had become frail in recent years but did not want to leave her home of 50 years to live with her children in another state. She missed her husband and had been depressed since his death 6 months before. Her depression often left her confused, and one evening she mistakenly took a double dose of one of her medications and became dizzy. On her way to bed, she fell down the steps and broke her hip. She spent 2 months in the hospital but never

(continued on p. 6)

FIGURE 1.2
Leading Causes of Death by Age, 1987

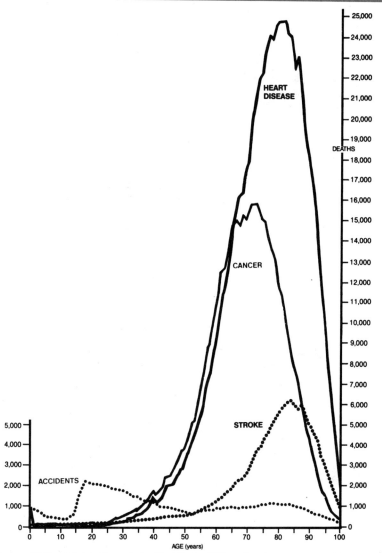

Source: National Safety Council, *Accident Facts*, 1990, p. 8.

Did You Know That . . .

In all developed countries, the leading cause of death for people aged 15 to 24 is motor vehicle accidents. Australia has the highest rate of male auto fatalities, with the United States coming in second, according to a Census Bureau report.

Heart disease, cancer, stroke, and accidents were the leading causes of death in the United States in 1987. This graph depicts the number of deaths attributed to these causes by age. Accidents were the leading cause of death from age 1 to 37. Persons age 18 suffered the greatest number of lives lost to accidents.

How People Died Accidentally in 1989

Type of accident and age of victim

	Death Total	Change from 1988	Death Rate[2]

All accidents

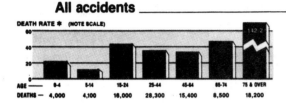

94,500   **– 2%**   **38.1**

The term "accidents" covers most deaths from injury and poisoning. Excluded are homicides, suicides, deaths for which none of these categories can be determined, and war deaths.

Motor-vehicle accidents

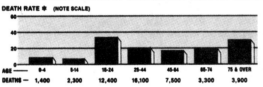

46,900   **– 4%**   **18.9**

Includes deaths involving mechanically or electrically powered highway-transport vehicles in motion (except those on rails), both on and off the highway or street.

Falls

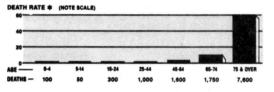

12,400   **+ 2%**   **5.0**

Includes deaths from falls from one level to another or on the same level. Excludes falls in or from transport vehicles, or while boarding or alighting from them.

Poisoning by solids and liquids

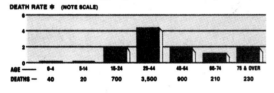

5,600   **+10%**   **2.3**

Includes deaths from drugs, medicines, mushrooms and shellfish, as well as commonly recognized poisons. Excludes poisonings from spoiled foods, salmonella, etc., which are classified as disease deaths.

Drowning

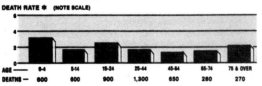

4,600   **0%**   **1.9**

Includes all drownings (work and nonwork) in boat accidents and those resulting from swimming, playing in the water, or falling in. Excludes drownings in floods and other cataclysms.

	Death Total	Change from 1988	Death Rate[2]

Fires, burns, and deaths associated with fires _____

4,400   -6%   1.8

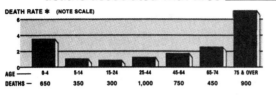

DEATH RATE * (NOTE SCALE)

AGE	0-4	5-14	15-24	25-44	45-64	65-74	75 & OVER
DEATHS	650	350	300	1,000	750	450	900

Includes death from fires, burns, and from injuries in conflagrations—such as asphyxiation, falls, and struck by falling objects. Excludes burns from hot objects or liquids.

Suffocation by ingested object _____

3,900   -3%   1.6

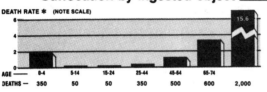

DEATH RATE * (NOTE SCALE)

AGE	0-4	5-14	15-24	25-44	45-64	65-74	
DEATHS	350	50	50	350	500	600	2,000

Includes deaths from accidental ingestion or inhalation of objects or food resulting in the obstruction of respiratory passages.

Firearms _____

1,600   +7%   0.6

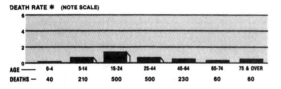

DEATH RATE * (NOTE SCALE)

AGE	0-4	5-14	15-24	25-44	45-64	65-74	75 & OVER
DEATHS	40	210	500	500	230	60	60

Includes deaths in firearms accidents principally in recreational activities or on home premises. Excludes deaths from explosive material or in war operations.

Poisoning by gases and vapors _____

900   0%   0.4

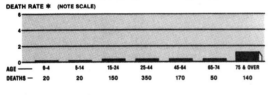

DEATH RATE * (NOTE SCALE)

AGE	0-4	5-14	15-24	25-44	45-64	65-74	75 & OVER
DEATHS	20	20	150	350	170	50	140

Mostly carbon monoxide due to incomplete combustion, involving cooking and heating equipment and standing motor vehicles. Excludes deaths in conflagrations, or associated with transport vehicles in motion.

All other types _____

14,200   -3%   5.7

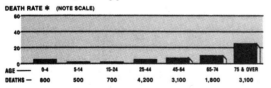

DEATH RATE * (NOTE SCALE)

AGE	0-4	5-14	15-24	25-44	45-64	65-74	75 & OVER
DEATHS	800	500	700	4,200	3,100	1,800	3,100

Most important types included are: medical complications, air transport, machinery, mechanical suffocation, and struck by falling object.

*Deaths per 100,000 population in each age group.

[2]Deaths per 100,000 population.

FIGURE 1.3

Accidents vs. Natural Disasters as a Cause of Death

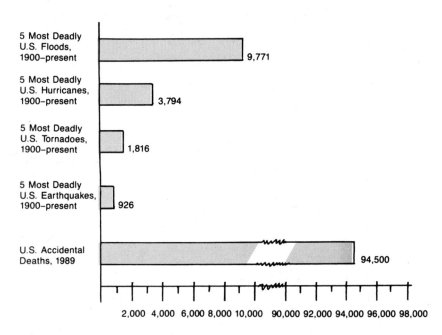

Source: Based on data from National Safety Council, *Accident Facts*, 1990, pp. 4, 5, 15.

Although floods, earthquakes, and other types of natural disasters are much feared, they kill far fewer people than accidents. In fact, the total number of people who died in natural disasters of all types in this country since 1900 is smaller by far than the number of people killed by accidents in 1989.

regained her full strength or mobility and had to be placed in a nursing home. She never lived independently again, and her home had to be sold to help cover her medical expenses.

Marion was cooking dinner for her family and watching 15-month-old Joshua when she received a phone call. She tried to keep an eye on the toddler as she talked but became momentarily distracted by the news that her sister's husband had received a promotion. After she hung up the phone, she noticed that Joshua was not around. In the few moments she had been on the phone, the boy had opened the screen door, wandered into the backyard, and fallen into the built-in pool. His mother revived him with

(continued on p. 8)

Some 57 million people in the United States are injured every year, and the annual price tag for these injuries has soared to $180 billion in 1988, according to a study by researchers at the University of California, San Francisco, and the Johns Hopkins School of Public Health.

"Injury is a major public health problem in the United States, striking one in four Americans a year," says Dorothy P. Rice, a researcher at the UCSF Institute for Health and Aging and a professor in the UCSF School of Nursing's Department of Social and Behavioral Sciences.

National Price Tag For Injuries Soars

The study was produced for the National Highway Traffic Safety Administration and the Centers for Disease Control by Rice and Ellen J. MacKenzie of the Johns Hopkins Injury Prevention Center.

Some data show that strategies can be used now to reduce the number of severe injuries, Rice said. The potential savings could be in the billions of dollars.

The following are among the study's findings:

• In 1985, 143,000 people in the United States died from injuries. For children and young adults under age 45, injury is the leading cause of death.

• Falls are the leading cause of injury, accounting for one third of fatal injuries. Firearms are the second largest cause of fatal injury.

• Some 2.3 million of the injuries in 1985 were serious enough to require hospitalization. The other 54 million injuries did not require hospitalization, but some form of medical care was needed.

• Injury is the leading cause of disability; Americans spent 127 million days in bed because of injuries in 1987.

• Fatalities represent less than 1% of all injuries but $31% of the total cost.

• The annual costs for medical care for injuries are $45 billion. This includes hospital and nursing home care, physician services, drugs, and rehabilitation.

Despite the high incidence and cost of injury, relatively little is spent on injury research, according to Rice and MacKenzie. Some $160 million in federal funds were spent on injury-related research in 1987. In comparison, $1.4 billion were spent by the National Institutes of Health on cancer research and $930 million on studies of heart disease.

The study concludes that investments in prevention could save the national economy billions of dollars each year and recommends that more money be directed to injury prevention research.

Source: *Healthline*, April 1991, p. 13.

Did You Know That . . .

Each and every day, an average of 170,000 Americans obtain medical services for injuries resulting from non-fatal accidents.

artificial respiration, but he suffered brain injuries that left him in a **vegetative** state.

Dave's expertise as a finish carpenter was well recognized in the construction firm where he worked. When a precision job was needed, Dave could always be counted on to do it. Not only was he skilled, but he was fast. Younger workers admired and often imitated the way he removed safety attachments from power tools in order to work faster. It was not surprising, therefore, when his boss asked him to work an extra shift one night to complete the trimming of a restaurant that had to be finished within the next 24 hours.

When Dave's second consecutive 8-hour shift ended with work still left to be done, his boss asked for a few more hours. Tired but eager to earn the double overtime pay, Dave agreed. Two hours later, bleary-eyed from exhaustion, Dave ran his right hand into the radial arm saw blade, slicing off 4 fingers. Attempts were made to re-attach the fingers in emergency surgery, but they were unsuccessful. Dave never worked again as a finish carpenter and, lacking other skills, entered the ranks of the permanently unemployed.

Accidents similar to the fictionalized incidents described above occur every day in the United States, claiming 95,000 lives a year and causing permanent **disability** to another 350,000 persons. While the emotional cost of these accidents to the families involved cannot be measured, the dollar cost to our economy is estimated at $148.5 billion a year in medical expenses and lost income. [1]

There is no doubt that accidents are a major health problem in America. They are the leading cause of death and disability for people between the ages of one and 44. In older groups only heart disease, cancer, stroke, and diabetes take a greater toll.

Accidents are so commonplace, however, that they often do not receive the attention that their seriousness deserves. They are often viewed as less threatening than natural disasters such as earthquakes, tornadoes, hurricanes, volcanic eruptions, and floods. Yet the total number of casualties resulting from the 5 largest natural disasters of all types over the last 25 years is less than half the number of deaths caused by accidents in a single year. Twice as many people are killed every year in accidents as were killed in the entire Vietnam War. In just 4 years, accidents kill as many Americans as were killed in all of World War II. [2]

The injury picture is no less troublesome. Around the country today are scores of **rehabilitation centers** that specialize in caring for patients with brain or spinal injuries. Brain-injured

Artificial respiration: The rhythmic forcing of air in and out of the lungs of a person who is not breathing.

Vegetative: A state in which one is unable to respond to external stimuli.

Disability: Any bodily or mental impairment, particularly one that results in inability to pursue an occupation or activity.

Rehabilitation centers: Facilities designed to help injured people by providing training and instruction in how to function with or recover from the effects of injury.

(continued on p. 11)

Costs of Accidents in 1989

Accidents in which deaths or disabling injuries occurred, together with vehicle accidents and fires, cost the nation in 1989, at least

$148.5 billion

Motor-vehicle accidents .... **$72.2 billion**
This cost figure includes wage loss, medical expense, insurance administration cost, and insured property damage from moving motor-vehicle accidents. Not included are the cost of public agencies such as police and fire departments, courts, indirect losses to employers of off-the-job accidents to employees, the value of cargo losses in commercial vehicles, and damages awarded in excess of direct losses. Fire damage to parked motor-vehicles is not included here but is distributed to the other classes.

Work accidents .... **$48.5 billion**
This cost figure includes wage loss, medical expense, insurance administration cost, fire loss, and an estimate of indirect costs arising out of work accidents. Not included is the value of property damage other than fire loss, and indirect loss from fires.

Home accidents .... **$18.2 billion**
This cost figure includes wage loss, medical expense, health insurance administration cost, and fire loss. Not included are the costs of property damage other than fire loss, and the indirect cost to employers of off-the-job accidents to employees.

Public accidents .... **$12.5 billion**
This cost figure includes wage loss, medical expense, health insurance administration cost, and fire loss. Not included are the costs of property damage other than fire loss, and the indirect cost to employers of off-the-job accidents to employees.

1989 accident cost components
TOTAL—ALL ACCIDENTS .... **$148.5 billion**

These costs include:

Wage loss .... **$37.7 billion**
Since, theoretically, a worker's contribution to the wealth of the nation is measured in terms of wages, then the total of wages lost due to accidents provides a measure of this lost productivity.

For nonfatal injuries, actual wage losses are used; for fatalities and permanent disabilities, the figure used is the present value of all future earnings lost.

Medical expense .... **$23.7 billion**
Doctor fees, hospital charges, the cost of medicines, ambulance and emergency medical services, and future medical costs incurred as the result of accidental injuries are included.

Insurance administration cost .... **$28.4 billion**
This is the difference between premiums paid to insurance companies and claims paid out by them; it is their cost of doing business and is a part of the accident cost total. Claims paid by insurance companies are not identified separately, as every claim is compensation for losses such as wages, medical expenses, property damage, etc., which are included in other categories above and below. *Not* included are administrative costs of health maintenance organizations and property damage claims in home and public accidents.

Property damage in motor-vehicle accidents ..... **$26.8 billion**
Includes the value of insured property damage to vehicles from moving motor-vehicle accidents. The damage is valued at the cost to repair the vehicle or the market value of the vehicle when damage exceeds its market value. The cost of minor damage (such as scratches or dents incurred while parking) is considered part of the normal wear and tear to vehicles and is not included.

Fire loss .... **$9.4 billion**
Includes losses from building fires of $8.1 billion and from nonbuilding fires, of $1.3 billion. By class of accident these totals break down as follows: building–work $2.9 billion, home $4.4 billion, public $0.8 billion; nonbuilding–work $0.6 billion, home $0.2 billion, public $0.5 billion.

Indirect loss from work accidents .... **$22.5 billion**
This is the money value of time lost by noninjured workers. Includes time spent filling out accident reports, giving first aid to injured workers, and time lost due to production slowdowns. This loss is conservatively estimated as equal to the sum of lost wages, medical expenses, and insurance administration cost of work accidents.

National Safety Council estimates. Cost estimates are not comparable with those of previous years. As additional or more precise data become available, they are used from that year forward, but previously estimated figures are not revised.

Source: National Safety Council, *Accident Facts, 1990*, pp. 2–3.

FIGURE 1.4
Trends in Accidental Death Rates

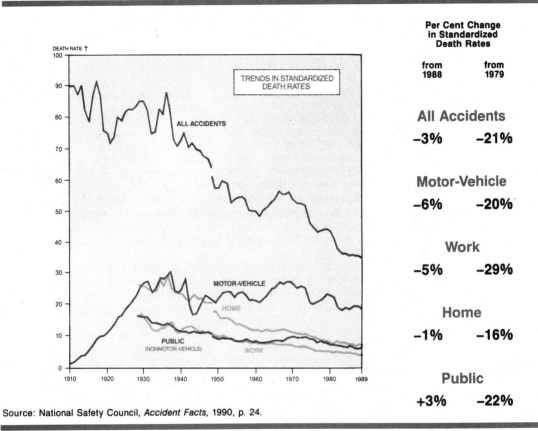

Per Cent Change
In Standardized
Death Rates

	from 1988	from 1979
All Accidents	**–3%**	**–21%**
Motor-Vehicle	**–6%**	**–20%**
Work	**–5%**	**–29%**
Home	**–1%**	**–16%**
Public	**+3%**	**–22%**

Source: National Safety Council, *Accident Facts*, 1990, p. 24.

Between 1912 and 1989, the overall accidental death rate in the United States declined by 54 percent. The reduction would have been even greater except for a six-fold increase in the motor vehicle death rate. The death rates depicted above have been adjusted (standardized) to the age distribution of the U.S. population in 1940.

patients struggle to relearn simple tasks such as walking, talking, and self-care in therapy programs that can stretch into years. Patients paralyzed because of spinal injuries have to learn how to begin life again from a wheelchair. These patients learn how to cope, but they face lives of curtailed opportunity, lost potential, and ongoing health difficulties. The majority of patients in these programs are accident victims. If automobile accidents alone

(continued on p. 15)

Gradually and with little fanfare, anxious Americans have reduced one measure of risk in their daily lives: In the last decade, the death rate from accidents has dropped 21 percent as more cautious conduct has been institutionalized in law and custom.

The figures, released in August [1990] by the National Safety Council, a Congressionally chartered group in Chicago whose statistics are considered authoritative,

Fatal Accidents Are Down

include a 20 percent decline in the rate of motor vehicle deaths, which account for nearly half of all accidental deaths. The biggest drop was among drivers 15 to 24 years old.

The death rate from accidents at work, like motor vehicle crashes and falls, dropped 29 percent. The death rate for public accidents, which include falls, drownings and plane crashes, declined 22 percent, while the death rate from accidents in the home, like falls, poisonings and fires, fell 16 percent. If not for a significant increase in accidental fatal drug overdoses, the death rate in the home would have fallen much further.

No Single Reason

Indeed, more progress was made in accident prevention in the 1980's than in any other decade in this century, according to the council. The 87-year-old nonprofit organization, set up to educate people about safety, has 300 employees and an annual budget of $27 million in private financing.

While the drop in the accident death rate reflects the lowered odds of an individual's risk in a given year, the overall number of accidents has also fallen, despite the growth in population. The total annual number of fatal accidents fell from 105,312 in 1979 to 94,500 in 1989. The risk of dying in a car accident is lower now than at any other time since the 1920's, although the abandonment of a nationwide 55 mile-per-hour speed limit has started to increase the hazards again.

Officials at the council are reluctant to ascribe the national decline to any particular factor, saying the requisite studies have never been done. "You can't put your finger on any one thing," said Nina Moroz, manager of the group's home safety programs.

But changed attitudes and regulations clearly account for some of the decline in fatal accidents, which rank as the fourth leading cause of death, after heart disease, cancer and strokes.

Safety Laws and Campaigns

Campaigns against drunken driving have reduced deaths from auto accidents, and a similar effort directed at boaters may be reducing the risk of drowning. "A lot of attention has been focused on alcohol and boating," said Albert Marmo, executive director of the National Boating Safety Advisory Council. Half of all boating deaths involve alcohol.

A large decline in fire deaths in the early 1980's is partly credited to widespread use of smoke detectors. But a big drop in deaths from 1988 through 1989 is difficult to explain. Smoke detectors could be a factor, but the change could also be linked to a national decline in the percentage of smokers, said John Hall, director of fire analysis and research for the National Fire Protection Association in Boston. Cigarettes are the leading cause of fires in the home, where four in five fire deaths occur.

Accidental death rates vary widely from state to state. New York, which mandates smoke detectors in homes and was among the first states to require the use of seat belts and to institute tough laws against drunken drinking, has a lower accidental-death rate than any other state except Ohio. But safety experts cannot say why certain states are so much safer than others because so many factors, among them the quality of medical care, contribute to accidental death rates.

Many market researchers and academics attribute concern about safety to a population that is aging, is having fewer children and later in life, and is increasingly imbued with an urge to control overwhelming circumstances. Such people have propelled safety legislation, inspired the marketing of products like cars equipped with air bags and proved to be avid consumers for an emerging safety industry that provides personal alarms, no-slip bathmats, safer cutting boards and even a device that slips over shopping-cart handles, to keep babies from making contact with germs.

The vigilance has increased gradually, stemming at least in part from the consumer movement that took hold in the 1970's, championed by Ralph Nader. In the 1980's, campaigns against drunken driving and public smoking reinforced the notion that Americans could no longer impinge on the safety of others.

But while danger always makes news, the reduction of certain risks seems to go unnoticed and thus fails to make people more secure. Some experts believe Americans are becoming ever more nervous about a multitude of safety issues surrounding food, water, air and technology.

"There is a very high level of anxiety in the United States," said Leo J. Shapiro, Chairman of Leo J. Shapiro Associates in Chicago, a market research company. He believes this stems from the sense that individuals are responsible for both the bad and the good things that happen in their lives. They are less likely to blame fate than in the past, his research shows.

Fears Detached From Reality

Trying to avoid all risk, however may actually enhance anxiety. "If you're constantly taking measures, you increase the atmosphere of fear you're living in," said Richard A. Gordon, a professor of psychology at Bard College in Annendale-on-Hudson, N.Y., and a clinical psychologist in private practice.

In a risk-filled world, an individual's fears are likelier to reflect personal philosophy than external reality, said Aaron Wildavsky, a professor of political science and public policy at the University of California at Berkeley who has written several books on risk. Politically liberal egalitarians, he said, tend to fear technology. People who are hierarchical in their beliefs, like evangelical Christians or Mormons, are willing to be reassured by experts. Competitive individualists see risk as an opportunity.

"People's rating of danger is not affected by knowledge," said Professor Wildavsky. "The more you distrust institutions, the more fearful you are of the products of corporate capitalism."

But prescient capitalists have seen the fears about safety and figured out how to profit from them. A new chain called the Safety Zone has opened five outlets in the past year, one in Woodbridge, N.J., and plans to open dozens in 1991. It sells every imaginable safety device, from kits to test water for lead to baseballs that don't hurt. Melanie Franklin, a partner in the company with her husband, Anthony Lee, believes the Safety Zone helps people handle anxiety. Ms. Franklin, for instance, always carries a small alarm to scare off assailants. "For me, it's peace of mind," she said.

Nowhere is the push for safety more pronounced than in the marketing to parents. Sales of items in the Perfectly Safe Catalogue, which offers items like latches to keep cupboards shut and gates to prevent falls down stairs are growing 15 percent a month, said Jeanne E. Miller, vice president of the Duncan Hill Group, a direct marketer in North Canton, Ohio, that puts out the catalogue.

Five years ago, Michael Lerner started selling the "Baby on Board" signs that became ubiquitous in cars. Now his company, Safety 1st, Inc., in Chestnut Hill, Mass., has 75 products, partly inspired by changes in child rearing. "When I was growing up," said Mr. Lerner, "my mother was always there." Twenty years ago, he added, no state required that children ride in safety seats in cars. Now, all do.

Arnold Brown, a partner in Weiner, Edrich, Brown, a New York company that advises corporations about future trends, believes that safety is becoming the newest obsession of the baby boom generation, taking its place alongside fitness. The heightened concern for children's safety, he said, makes sense at a time of shrinking families. "If you lose your child now," he said, "you lose your family."

Source: Trish Hall, "Fatal Accidents Are Down As U.S. Becomes Vigilant," *New York Times*, 7 October 1990, pp. 1, 32.

were eliminated, the need for such services would shrink by as much as 50 percent. [3]

The high number of deaths and injuries is the bad news about accidents, but there is some good news as well. Many accidents are preventable. Accident causes can be identified and many can be controlled. If we analyze the accidents described at the beginning of this chapter, for instance, we can identify clear warning signs in each case. Statistically each victim was at a high risk of suffering the type of accident he or she experienced. A working knowledge of the most common accidents and the factors that lead to them could have helped these people take precautions.

HUMAN FACTORS

While each accident is unique in the sense that it happens to a particular person or persons at a specific time and place, certain factors are common to virtually all types of accident. The most important of these from a prevention standpoint are the human factors.

Attitudes

Most safety professionals agree that one of the most important causes of accidents is the attitude of the individual. An inclination to take risks and behave recklessly leads to accidents. Believing that safety precautions are a waste of time or that if an accident is going to occur there is little anyone can do to stop it are also examples of dangerous attitudes.

Emotions

Emotions such as depression, fear, anger, hatred, anxiety, and joy can lead to unpredictable behavior, which in turn can cause accidents. Emotional **stress** has also been correlated with accident-producing behavior. [4]

Habits

Habits are automatic responses to certain **stimuli**. They are formed through repeated experiences and do not involve conscious thought. Some habits, such as wearing a seat belt or riding a bicycle with the flow of traffic, promote safety. Other habits, such as drinking while driving, speeding, and not wearing proper protective gear, are unsafe practices that can result in accidental injury or death.

Stress: Any disruption, change, or adjustment in a person's mental, emotional, or physical well-being caused by an external stimulus, either physical or psychological.

Stimuli: Any external events or actions that prompt a response on the part of the individual who is exposed to them.

(continued on p. 18)

Some cold medications can impair a driver's ability in much the same way that alcohol would. One study showed that 50 milligrams of antihistamine has the same impact on a person as a blood alcohol level of 50 to 100 milligrams per 100 milliliters.

Mike had just left basketball practice. He was hungry, tired, and angry. The coach had just told him he would not start in Friday night's game.

Mike tramped through the rain to his car, opened the door, and dropped into the seat. Just as he started the car, his teammate Andy ran from the gym, waved his arms, and asked for a ride home. "Sure," said Mike. "Climb in."

How Accidental Are Accidents?

Streaks appeared on the dirty, grease-coated windshield as Mike turned on the wipers. "Stupid windshield wipers," grumbled Mike as he stomped on the accelerator and spun his wheels. The car raced down the wet side street as Mike angrily told Andy how he felt he had been cheated out of his starting spot. Suddenly a man appeared out of nowhere to cross at a crosswalk. Mike swerved to miss him and slid on the wet pavement, crashing into a tree. Both boys, neither of them protected by a seat belt, were thrown into the windshield and knocked unconscious.

The newspaper implied the weather was to blame for the accident, but was it? By definition, an accident is any unintentional and undesirable happening resulting in injury, death, or property damage, but most accidents can be prevented. Ninety percent of accidents are attributed to something a person does or does not do. Six percent are due to equipment failure and four percent to the environment.

The leading causes of accidental death for our population are:

- motor vehicle accidents
- falls
- drowning
- fires and burns
- suffocation
- poisoning by mouth
- firearm injuries
- gas poisoning

As in Mike's story, analysis of accidents often shows that either personal or physical factors led to the accident.

The Personal Factor
Personal factors are far more likely to cause accidents than are physical ones. They include stress, fatigue, age, lack of knowledge or skill, use of drugs, and attitude.
• **Stress**—When people are under stress, as Mike was, they often experience strong emotions that can interfere with concentration. Things such as changing weather conditions, a dirty windshield, or a person crossing the street might be overlooked if a person is angry. Anger is particularly dangerous because it distracts us from the task at hand, so it is wise, for example, to cool down before getting behind the wheel.
• **Fatigue**—When people are tired, as Mike was, they are less alert. They might risk dozing off or, at the very least, suffer from poor

coordination. Whether you are driving or doing something like swimming, alertness and coordination are important, so don't attempt difficult tasks when you're tired.

Different Hazards

• **Age**—At each age, there are slightly different hazards. There are more accidental deaths at age 18 than any other age. Why are the teen years so dangerous? First, because it is an age at which we are easily influenced by peers. A teen may be more likely to take dares and risks. In addition, young people may lack the experience in dealing with emergencies and may even lack the skill.

Very old people also have a higher incidence of accidents, like falling, because of a decrease in strength, flexibility, coordination, and vision. Some may be slower at making decisions a driver has to make.

• **Lack of knowledge or skill** may be a factor at any age. Not knowing the rules of the road would make an 18-year-old a dangerous driver. A 10-year-old may not know how to operate a lawn mower or be strong enough to maneuver it on an incline. Poor judgment can also stem from a lack of knowledge. A person who doesn't even consider wearing safety goggles when using power tools may not know that power tools often create missiles that can damage the eyes.

Still another example of this can be a failure to plan ahead. Going hiking at noon on a 72-degree day in a T-shirt and shorts could lead to disaster if you get lost and the temperature drops to 50 degrees at twilight.

Drugs to Blame

• **Drugs**—Alcohol is implicated in at least 50 percent of highway fatalities, fatal fires, drownings, and deaths at the workplace. If you know a little about drugs, you know that many of them can impair reflexes, perception, coordination, concentration, and judgment. Even over-the-counter drugs, such as cold medications, can make you sleepy and impair your coordination. Many teen drownings are related to the use of alcohol, as are boat accidents.

• **Attitude**—How you feel about what you are about to do has a lot to do with whether you will do it safely. An attitude of overconfidence can be one of the most dangerous attitudes to have. Mike probably felt he could drive on wet pavement as well as he could on dry, and at the same speed. No doubt, he also thought accidents only happen to other people; otherwise he would have put on his seat belt. When we neglect to use safety equipment, it may reflect an attitude that such precautions are unnecessary.

The Physical Factor

Physical factors may include weather, equipment failure, and even time of day or time of year. Some of these factors can be minimized by taking precautions. Consider these:

Did You Know That . . .

Drivers who haven't had enough sleep are danger-ous. Experts say a sleep-deprived person can nod off within the first 15 minutes of an auto trip, and is most likely to do so at midday.

• **Weather**—Mike, in a calmer mood, would probably have remembered that stopping distance is increased by wet pavement, and visibility is decreased by rain. Thus, he would have reduced his speed and cleaned his windshield. That doesn't stop the rain, but it does improve the ability to drive in it. Subconsciously, we are constantly making adjustments for the weather. Consider the way you walk on a dry sidewalk compared to an icy one. It's always wise, too, to listen to weather forecasts before boating, swimming, skiing, or even playing golf, so you can adjust to the environment.

• **Equipment failure**—Brakes can fail, tires can blow out, baseball bats can break, and electrical cords can become frayed. Even so, equipment failure is seldom responsible for accidents, especially if the equipment is maintained properly.

However, if equipment does fail, then a person needs to have a plan of action. Have you thought about how you would react if your brakes were to fail on a hill? You should think about it and then you might know to try the emergency brake.

We also need to actually *use* safety equipment. A baseball bat that breaks and hits a catcher is less likely to cause injury if the catcher is wearing a helmet, face mask, throat protector, chest protector, and shin guards.

• **Time of day or time of year**—Certain times of day are more dangerous than others. For example, driving at 1 A.M. on a Friday or Saturday night is more dangerous, from the standpoint of drunk drivers, than driving at 8 A.M. Monday morning. Night is more dangerous than day, due to poorer visibility, and rush hour may be a more dangerous time than others to drive because of heavy traffic, stress, and fatigue.

Give another thought to the personal and physical factors in Mike's accident. Of course, he would have avoided it if he could have. Could he have?

Source: Candy Purdy, *Current Health 2* (March 1990), pp. 18–19.

Lack of Skill or Knowledge

In certain situations, lacking the proper skill or knowledge for a task can result in an accident. This is especially true when performing a new task. It has been shown, for example, that beginning and unskilled motorcycle operators have very high accident rates. Inadequate knowledge has also been shown to be a factor in many workplace accidents, especially in workplaces where technical knowledge is required, such as in the use of electrical equipment, chemicals, and high-speed machines.

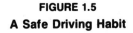

FIGURE 1.5
A Safe Driving Habit

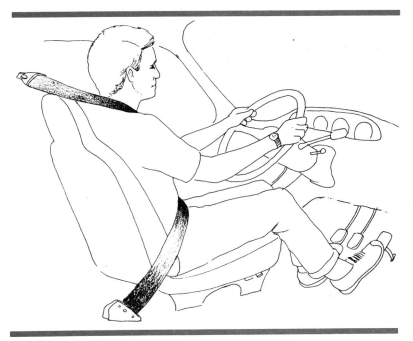

Numerous research studies indicate that lap and shoulder safety belts, when used, reduce the risk of fatal or serious injury to front-seat occupants by between 40 and 55 percent.

Alcohol and Drug Abuse

The use of alcohol and other drugs (including prescription medications when used inappropriately) is a tremendous accident-causing factor. Tasks such as driving, which are usually not hazardous if the driver is sober, become downright dangerous if the driver's vision and reaction time, as well as his or her judgment, are affected by a **psychoactive** substance. Alcohol and drug abuse can cause accidents at home and on the job, as well as on the road.

Failure to Use Safety Equipment

Seat belts in automobiles and safety devices on power tools are examples of equipment that can prevent accidents or lessen their severity. Failure to use them increases accident risk unnecessarily.

Psychoactive: Having the potential to alter mood or behavior.

FIGURE 1.6
Accidental Poisoning

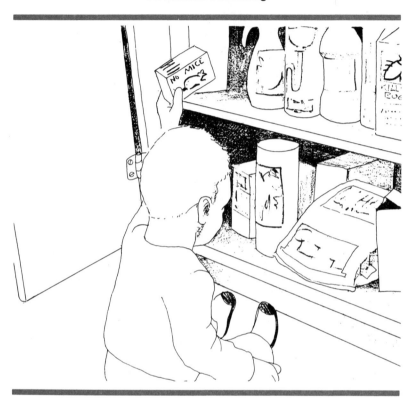

Infants and toddlers are curious about everything and will put almost anything in their mouths, no matter how it tastes. Household cleaners, pesticides, and other toxic substances should be stored in a locked cabinet, preferably out of reach of the young child.

Failure to Supervise

Children, especially those under the age of 5, are often incapable of knowing about or applying safety precautions, so adults must do it for them. In only a few moments of unsupervised time, toddlers can easily endanger themselves. Older adults may suffer physical or mental disabilities that leave them unable to ensure their own safety in all situations. Some elderly patients may need constant supervision, or they may benefit from additional safety measures, such as paging devices that connect directly to an emergency operator.

(continued on p. 23)

Make Your Home Poison-Proof

Fears about accidental home poisonings are well-founded. The U.S. Food and Drug Administration estimates that about three-fifths of non-fatal home poisonings happen to youngsters less than 5 years old.

Hundreds of thousands of children suffer from non-fatal poisonings each year. In addition, a disturbing number of adults—about 3,000 each year—die from accidental ingestion or inhalation of toxic solids, liquids, or gases. It's estimated that about 90% of accidental poisonings occur in the home.

In the sections ahead, Dr. Regine Aronow, director of the Poison Control Center for the Children's Hospital of Michigan in Detroit, describes how to prevent an accidental poisoning in the home.

When your children are small, always look for child-resistant packaging. Remember, though, *child-resistant* doesn't necessarily mean *child-proof*. Containers that are child-resistant are designed to keep out 80% of children less than 4 years old. But that still leaves 20% of children unprotected.

Never use old food containers to mix and store non-food products. Don't mix pesticides in a gallon milk jar, and never use soft-drink bottles to hold paint thinner.

Prevention is key, Aronow says. The best way to prevent accidental home poisonings is unrelenting vigilance. "Safe homes take hard work and a real awareness that one mistake could be deadly. But as the caretakers of young children, the responsibility is ours."

Here are some potential poisons to look out for:

Cleaning Materials: Many of the following products are highly toxic and should be stored away from food products. Also, be careful not to put pesticides, such as roach killers and ant killers, in places where children and toddlers could find them. Many such products are sweetened to attract bugs, and if kids get at them, the products can do real harm.

- Dishwasher detergents (liquid and granular)
- Laundry detergents
- Bleaches
- Ammonia
- Rust removers
- Liquid and crystal toilet bowl cleaners
- Furniture polish (especially oil-based)
- Lamp oils
- Aluminum siding cleaners
- Paint thinners
- Brush cleaners
- Paint strippers.

Medications: Be careful with prescriptions and over-the-counter products. Don't take medication in front of small children; they tend to imitate adults and could accidentally ingest a poisonous substance. Store medications away from food products. Clean out your medicine cabinet periodically and dispose of unneeded medicines simply by flushing them down the toilet. Keep the following out of sight and locked up:

- Cough and cold remedies
- Aspirin and aspirin substitutes
- Vitamin and mineral supplements
- Folk medicines and herbal preparations.

Vitamin and mineral supplements are packaged in child-size dosages and offered in colors, shapes, and flavors designed to appeal to young people. These products are often kept on the breakfast table or kitchen counter for convenience, Aronow says. Once kids get into them, they eat them like candy. And many supplements contain iron, which can be a serious poison when taken in tablet form.

Personal Care Products: Parents are often unaware of the danger posed to children by cosmetics and beauty aids, so they leave them out on the dresser or bathroom vanity.

Many personal care products contain alcohol, and a small amount can bring down the blood sugar level and endanger the child's brain. "Because a child's body mass is so small, it takes only a few swallows for the damage to be done," Aronow says.

Store these products properly:

- Cosmetics
- Beauty aids

- Nail polish removers
- Home permanent wave solutions
- Hair-conditioning products
- Rubbing alcohol
- Liniment
- Mouthwash
- After-shave lotions

Is Your Home Poison-Proof?

The following is a checklist of poisonous products found in the home. You should make sure that none of these products is within reach of children.

Kitchen
- [ ] medications
- [ ] drain cleaner—lye
- [ ] furniture polish
- [ ] powder and liquid detergent
- [ ] cleanser and scouring powder
- [ ] metal cleaner
- [ ] ammonia
- [ ] oven cleaner
- [ ] glass cleaner
- [ ] multivitamin with iron
- [ ] carpet and upholstery cleaners
- [ ] plants

Bedroom
- [ ] sleeping pills
- [ ] jewelry cleaner
- [ ] cosmetics—personal care products
- [ ] perfume

Laundry
- [ ] bleach
- [ ] soap and detergent
- [ ] disinfectant
- [ ] rust remover
- [ ] spot remover

Closet, Attic, Storage Places
- [ ] ant, mouse, rat poisons
- [ ] moth balls and sprays

Bathroom
- [ ] aspirin and nonaspirin fever and pain medications
- [ ] all drugs and pills
- [ ] drain cleaner—lye

- [ ] iron pills
- [ ] permanent wave solutions
- [ ] insect repellants
- [ ] creams and ointments
- [ ] nail polish and remover
- [ ] suntan lotion
- [ ] shampoo, lotion to kill lice and scabies mites
- [ ] shaving lotion, cologne, and perfume
- [ ] toilet bowl cleaner
- [ ] hair remover and hair streightener
- [ ] pine oil and bath oil
- [ ] rubbing alcohol
- [ ] boric acid
- [ ] fluoride drops

Garage, Basement, Workshop
- [ ] lye
- [ ] kerosene
- [ ] windshield washer solvent
- [ ] bug killer
- [ ] gasoline
- [ ] lighter fluid
- [ ] turpentine
- [ ] paint remover and thinner
- [ ] paint
- [ ] weed killer
- [ ] fertilizer
- [ ] anti-freeze

General
- [ ] flaking paint
- [ ] repainted toys
- [ ] button batteries
- [ ] pet medications and care products
- [ ] glues

Purse
- [ ] all drugs and pills

- Colognes
- Bonded fingernail removers.

Pet Care Products: When you use sprays or bug bombs to get rid of fleas, be careful that the fallout doesn't land on stacks of diapers or baby clothes. Wear rubber gloves and wash off table-tops and food preparation surfaces after spraying. Look out for:

- Pet medications (such as flea collars)
- Heartworm pills (store separately from your medications to prevent confusion).

Carbon Monoxide Fumes: "No single substance causes more accidental home poisonings than carbon monoxide," Aronow cautions. Your furnace and chimney need checking every year, along with your hot-water heater and any other gas appliances, to ensure against leaking fumes. And never run gasoline or fuel-powered motors inside the house; they can cause carbon monoxide buildup.

House Plants: House plants are the leading source of poisonings to children under 1 year of age. Keep plants off the floor and away from a child's reach, and watch out for plants that dangle overhead where kids can get to them.

Parents also need to take great care when using plant fertilizers and pesticides. They can be highly poisonous when absorbed through the skin during everyday use.

Plants from tropical regions, such as oleander, can be highly toxic. Plants with seeds (castor beans and rosary peas) are also dangerous. Stay away from wild-cherry wood, which can cause cyanide poisoning.

Car Care Products: Store and lock up automotive products preferably outside your home. Don't make the mistake of using car care products, such as windshield washer solvent, to clean the windows or other surfaces in your house. The following products pose a danger:

- Radiator antifreeze
- Windshield washer solvent
- Gas line antifreeze
- Brake and transmission fluids
- Whitewall cleaners.

Call for Help: Keep the phone number of the regional poison control center posted on your telephone. If you suspect that someone has been exposed to a dangerous substance, separate the person from the poison and call the center immediately for proper instruction.

Be Prepared: For every child in your home under the age of 6, keep a 1-ounce bottle of ipecac syrup.

This substance is available from your pharmacist and is used to empty the stomach. But never use ipecac without first consulting your physician or local poison center.

Source: Cathie Rategan, *Family Safety and Health* (Winter 1989–1990), pp. 22–23, and "Guide to Poison Prevention," Children's Hospital of Michigan, Poison Control Center, Detroit, Michigan.

Environmental Factors

Of course, not all accidents result solely from human error. Natural hazards such as snow, rain, dust, sleet, and fog increase the likelihood of accidents, especially in motor vehicles. In addition, man-made hazards can pose a danger. Many industrial jobs use large and complex machines. Although many of these have safety features, they are still a potential cause of accidents. Finally, poor working conditions and poor housekeeping are factors in many industrial and home accidents.

(continued on p. 25)

Did You Know That . . .

In 1988, 12,000 children had to go to hospital emergency rooms because of shopping cart accidents, usually with head injuries caused by falling out of the cart. Safety harnesses on carts help prevent such injuries.

Injuries are not accidents, says Vernon Houk, MD, an assistant surgeon general in the Public Health Service and director of the CDC's Center for Environmental Health and Injury Control in Atlanta, Ga.

Houk fines staff members 25 cents any time they utter the word "accident."

"He rightly argues that the word implies something is unpredictable, that there's no pattern to it," says Mark Rosenberg, MD, director of the center's Division of Injury Epidemiology and Control.

Preventive Medicine Extends to Injuries, Too

He vividly recalls having to dig for change in front of one of the top officials of the Department of Health and Human Services—"the assistant secretary for health. I used That Word, and he [Houk] stopped me dead in my tracks and asked for his quarter."

Rosenberg paid up because he agrees that the biggest barrier to reducing the incidence of injury is the "notion that things are just accidents you can't do anything about."

In truth, injuries are very predictable, says Houk, and "subject to the same epidemiology as infectious disease." Injuries are the number one killer of Americans younger than 45 years, and for all ages they are the leading cause of years of potential life lost (*Journal of the American Medical Association, JAMA*, 1989; 262: 2195). Fully 50% are preventable, "yet we do very little about it," Houk says.

Injury accounts for more years of life lost than cancer and cardiovascular disease put together. However, the amount spent on research is virtually the inverse of their incidence.

Until 2 years ago, Congress made no appropriation for injury studies at the CDC. Now, there is a $20-million program, which is still "peanuts," Houk contends, considering that injury takes 140,000 lives and costs $180 billion each year, accounting for one eighth of all hospital days and one third of all visits to physicians' offices.

There is a tremendous amount to be gained by developing effective interventions and showing that they work," says Rosenberg. "We're not supporting injury research at the level needed to catch up," he says.

The center's approach is to "try to understand the patterns behind types of injuries. Once the pattern is understood, they become quite predictable and suggest interventions," he says.

For example, studying youth suicides revealed that they do not occur in depressed persons as commonly believed, but in the "impulsive, the ones who get into trouble in school or with the police, who are angry and upset," he says.

Similarly, fire-related deaths—when "people in dilapidated housing use space heaters near incendiary material—are not accidents." Neither are poisonings when chemicals are left where children play, nor traffic deaths when people drive drunk, says Rosenberg.

Physicians can practice "a number of interventions directly with their patients," he adds. They should "ask about seat belts, child restraints, and bike helmets, make darn sure patients don't drink and drive, and look for intentional violence, especially spouse abuse."

They "need to work with the criminal justice system, social services, educators, highway safety people, firemen, lawyers, and legislators to develop policy to put research findings into action."

Source: Paul Cotton, *Journal of the American Medical Association,* Vol. 263, No. 19, 16 May 1990, p. 2597.

This book will examine in much greater detail the factors that play a part in accidents on the highway, in the home, at the workplace, and in public areas. Some of these will seem self-evident. Others will be surprising. Finding out about all of them can help prevent unnecessary tragedy. Knowledge can lead to safety, although we will learn later that knowledge alone is not enough. A commitment to change behavior is also important, as we will see.

CHAPTER

2

Safety on the Road

ANYONE WHO WOULD LIKE to live to a ripe old age in America needs to learn about the greatest health hazard for young people. That hazard is motor vehicle accidents. Motor vehicle crashes involving automobiles, motorcycles, or bicycles are the leading cause of death for people under the age of 38. The death rate is especially high for those in the 15-to-24 age group, more of whom die from accidents than from all other causes combined. Motor vehicle accidents also take a high toll on older age groups; it remains one of the top 5 causes of death up to the age of 64. [1]

Setting out for a drive, however, is not like a turn of the roulette wheel; chance alone does not determine whether someone will be injured or killed. The vast majority of motor vehicle crashes are directly associated with behavior that every driver (young or old) can control. These include driving while under the influence of alcohol, driving too fast for conditions, and not using seat belts.

Simply by observing the following 3 rules, therefore, you can greatly reduce your risk of death or injury as a result of a motor vehicle accident:

1. Don't drink and drive!

2. Don't speed!

3. Always wear a seat belt!

(continued on p. 28)

Myths Versus Facts About Safety Belt Use

Adult motor-vehicle occupants unaccustomed to buckling up often cite one or more of the following "reasons."

Myth: Belts are needed only for long trips and high-speed expressway driving.

Fact: Eighty percent of serious and fatal injuries occur in cars traveling less than 40 mph. Fatalities involving nonbelted occupants have been recorded at speeds as low as 12 mph. Conversely, there were no fatalities to belted occupants in a 28,000-vehicle study with speeds up to 60 mph. Seventy-five percent of serious and fatal injuries occur less than 25 miles from home.

Myth: Belts trap occupants in their vehicles, especially in cases of fire or submersion.

Fact: Less than one half of 1% of all injury-producing collisions involve fire or submersion. But even if fire or submersion does occur, wearing a safety belt can save a life. The unrestrained occupant will be slammed into the dashboard or windshield and knocked unconscious, and will therefore be unable to extricate himself or herself. Belts keep occupants unhurt and alert. Also, an unrestrained occupant rendered unconscious could block exit paths of other occupants.

Myth: It is better to be thrown clear of the vehicle.

Fact: A person is about 25 times more likely to be fatally injured if ejected from the vehicle than if inside and buckled up. Ejection can result not only in landing on unforgiving pavement but also in hitting other lethal roadside objects, scraping along the ground, or being crushed by one's own or another vehicle.

Myth: Occupants can brace themselves adequately in a crash.

Fact: The forces involved in even a low-speed crash make it impossible for anyone to avoid contact with the vehicle interior, which ultimately results in injury. At the moderate speed of 30 mph, an auto collision would throw occupants forward with a force equal to 30 times their body weight. Also, one out of four serious in-vehicle injuries is caused by occupants being thrown against each other.

Myth: Good drivers do not cause crashes.

Fact: First, the primary purpose of the safety belt is to protect against injury after the crash, and good drivers are equally vulnerable. Second, no driver can control the other. Considering that 50% of all fatal car crashes involve a drinking driver, a good driver cannot depend only on his or her own safe driving. Third, safety belts can make good drivers better. A belted driver will avoid fatigue and will have more control over the vehicle in emergencies. Finally, even good drivers can make sudden stops. In such situations, occupants are kept in place and protected against contact with the vehicle interior or with other occupants.

Myth: Safety belts don't work. They hang loose or do not lock up when pulled.

Fact: Late-model cars are equipped with a one-piece lap-shoulder belt that has been deliberately designed to allow freedom of movement as needed. This engineering advance answers the earlier argument that belts were confining and did not allow for easy access to necessary vehicle instruments. When needed, an inertial device locks the safety belt in place and keeps the occupants from making contact with the vehicle interior or from being partially or totally ejected.

Myth: Belts cause injuries.

Fact: Injuries due to belts have been reported. In these rare situations, however, either the belt was inappropriately worn or the crash was so severe that the occupants would have been seriously or fatally injured if not belted. Also, a belt-induced injury occurs to a part of the body better able to withstand the pressure exerted by the belt than the forces of the crash. There is no evidence to suggest that, without intrusion or some other compromising factor, safety belts by themselves generate life-threatening injuries.

Source: *The Safety Belt Proponent's Guide,* published by the Highway Users Federation and the Automotive Safety Foundation, reprinted in *Healthline,* October 1989.

DRINKING AND DRIVING

Despite greatly increased efforts in the last decade to stimulate public awareness of the dangers of drinking while driving, the number of alcohol-related accidents has decreased only slightly. Twenty-four thousand people still die annually in alcohol-related crashes (slightly less than half of the total motor vehicle accident fatalities). If accident rates continue at their present levels, more than 50 percent of all Americans will be involved in an alcohol-related accident in their lifetimes. [2]

One reason public awareness campaigns do not work very well is that many drivers believe it cannot happen to them. Even responsible drivers are often unaware of basic facts about the effects of alcohol on their ability to drive safely. For this reason it is important to go beyond simple slogans such as "Don't drink and drive," by asking and answering questions such as the following:

Question Number 1: *How does alcohol affect driving ability?*

A brief answer is, in many ways. In a series of studies, drivers were tested to see how well they responded to an emergency that required them to put on their brakes and make a quick turn in a simulated accident-avoidance maneuver. Drivers who passed this test easily before drinking were unable to do so after only 2 or 3 drinks. Reaction time for both braking and turning was seriously impaired.

Alcohol can also affect a driver's reaction to bright lights. At night when a driver faces the headlights of oncoming traffic, he or she is blinded momentarily until his or her pupils have time to become smaller in order to decrease the intensity of light. When reaction time is normal, this instant of blindness is hardly noticeable and does not interfere with driving. Studies have shown, however, that after drinking alcohol, the pupils react to light much more slowly, so the period of blindness is longer—lasting up to 15 seconds. To get an idea of how long this is, try closing your eyes for a slow count of 15 and imagine driving that long while blinded.

Peripheral vision: The ability to see objects and images on the outer fringes of the visual range.

In addition, alcohol narrows the range of a driver's **peripheral vision**. The driver can see what is straight ahead but not persons, cars, intersections, and movements to the side.

Sedative: A drug or agent that has calming effects on the nervous system.

Finally, drinking affects judgment and can cause sleepiness. Good driving continuously requires the ability to make sensible decisions based on sound reasoning. Alcohol dulls the parts of the brain that control good judgment and sound decisions. It is also a **sedative** with the same chemical composition as **ether**, the first

Ether: A colorless liquid once widely used as a general anesthetic; full name, diethyl ether.

FIGURE 2.1
It Can Happen to You

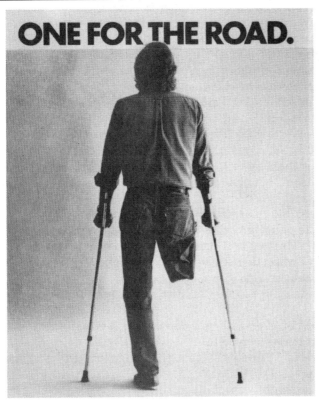

ONE FOR THE ROAD.

**Drink and drive, and you may lose something
on the way home from the party.**

Source: Reader's Digest Foundation.

general anesthetic, which was widely used until the 1930s. Although a drinker may feel stimulated when he or she first starts drinking, the sedative effects soon take over, causing sleepiness. A drowsy driver lacks the alertness and concentration to drive safely.

Question Number 2: *How much alcohol does it take to affect driving behavior?*

Alcohol has **anesthetic** properties that begin to take effect with the first drink. Driving behavior, consequently, begins to

Anesthetic: A substance that produces a loss of sensation.

decline from the very first sip. Studies have shown, for instance, that a person who has had only 4 drinks in one hour is 4 times as likely to be involved in a fatal accident as someone who has not been drinking. And alcohol can fool—it takes away from the driver's ability to judge his or her own performance. Most drivers are unaware of the subtle decline in their reaction time, alertness, and concentration that comes with a few drinks. They think they are doing fine right up to the moment of the accident.

Question Number 3: *How much does the chance of a fatal accident increase as drinking increases?*

After consuming 5 drinks in an hour, a driver is 7 times more likely to be involved in a fatal accident. A driver who has consumed 7 drinks in an hour is 25 times more likely to be involved in such an accident. Consuming 10 drinks in one hour increases the risk to 100 times the normal level.

Question Number 4: *Are the drunk driving laws keeping our roadways safe?*

Even though arrests of drunk drivers have gone up in recent years, the police are able to catch only a small fraction of those actually drinking and driving. Experts estimate that a person will drive while drunk (over the legal limit) 77 times before ever getting caught. [3]

In addition, recent statistics showed the following:

• One out of every 50 cars driving on the roadway is likely to have a drunk driver. [4]
• In the evening on weekends, that number goes up to one in 10 drivers.
• After midnight, especially at times when bars are closing, even a larger percentage are drunk.

Question Number 5: *Are most alcohol-related accidents caused by alcoholics?*

Only 10 percent of the population of drivers are alcoholics. Although they constitute a serious part of the drunk-driving problem in this country, many accidents are caused by persons who are not **addicted** to alcohol but instead are social drinkers or infrequent abusers of alcohol. Every person who drinks alcohol has the potential to cause an alcohol-related accident and needs to take precautions.

Question Number 6: *Are drivers the only ones who need to worry about drinking and driving?*

Although the majority of the victims of drunk-driving crashes are the drunk drivers themselves, 20 percent of those

Addicted: Psychologically or physiologically dependent on a chemical substance.

FIGURE 2.2
Approximate Blood Alcohol Concentration

Drinks	Body Weight in Pounds								
	100	120	140	160	180	200	220	240	
1	.04	.03	.03	.02	.02	.02	.02	.02	Possibly
2	.08	.06	.05	.05	.04	.04	.03	.03	Influenced
3	.11	.09	.08	.07	.06	.06	.05	.05	
4	.15	.12	.11	.09	.08	.08	.07	.06	
5	.19	.16	.13	.12	.11	.09	.09	.08	Under the
6	.22	.19	.16	.14	.13	.11	.10	.09	Influence
7	.26	.22	.19	.16	.15	.13	.12	.11	
8	.30	.25	.21	.19	.17	.15	.14	.13	
9	.34	.28	.24	.21	.19	.17	.15	.14	Intoxi-
10	.38	.31	.27	.23	.21	.19	.17	.16	cated

(Based on approximately 1 hour)

One drink equals: 1 oz. of 80 proof liquor; 12 oz. of beer; 4 oz. of wine (12% alcohol)
CAUTION: Many drinks have more than 1 oz. of alcohol.
Source: Connecticut Department of Transportation.

This chart shows the relationship between the number of drinks consumed by an adult and his or her body weight. Individuals may vary somewhat in their personal alcohol tolerance. Medications, health, and psychological conditions are also influential factors.

killed are passengers in the car of the drinker, and 17 percent are innocent drivers, passengers, and pedestrians not in the drunk driver's vehicle.

Question Number 7: *What myths do people believe about drinking and driving that are dangerous?*

There are many, but 3 seem to be most prevalent. Here they are, followed by the correct facts:

1) *Myth:* Drinking coffee, taking a cold shower, or exercising will sober you up quickly and allow you to drive.

Fact: None of these has any effect on **sobriety**. The only way alcohol leaves your body is as a result of being broken down into less harmful substances which are then eliminated at the rate of roughly 1 drink per hour. This is the maximum rate at which the liver, the organ primarily involved, can metabolize (process) alcohol. Only time will sober you up.

2) *Myth:* I will not get as drunk if I drink only beer or wine.

Fact: There is just as much alcohol in a bottle of beer as in a

(continued on p. 33)

Sobriety: A state of soberness – as opposed to intoxication.

Blood Alcohol Concentration

The healthy person can break down, or oxidize, approximately one drink per hour. Individual differences must be considered, such as weight, sex, drinking on an empty stomach, and so on. This amount offers a desired effect and helps prevent hangovers and/or allergic reactions.

GOING BEYOND ONE-DRINK-PER-HOUR

The following successive stages and effects of increasing alcohol consumption are calculated for a 150-pound male. Females of the same body weight will have slightly higher blood alcohol levels due to different body chemistry. Both men and women below 150 pounds should significantly lower their consumption.

Euphoria .02–.05 BAC*	=	1–2 drinks/hour or 3 drinks/2 hours or 4 drinks/3 hours

*BAC - Blood Alcohol Content

With initial doses of alcohol there is only a slight decrease in brain activity. You feel somewhat relaxed, social, or congenial.

Excitement .05–.08 BAC	=	3–4 drinks/hour or 5 drinks/2 hours or 6 drinks/3 hours

As you drink more, brain activity is further decreased, producing a loss of normal inhibitions. This is often mistaken for stimulation, but in fact, alcohol is depressing the brain centers responsible for restraining excessive behaviors, a function needed for routine judgment. This level of consumption can increase aggression and stress in emotional situations and can [a]ffect other activities, such as safe driving.

Confusion .09–.15 BAC	=	5–6 drinks/hour or 7 drinks/2 hours or 8 drinks/3 hours

This much alcohol produces intoxication. Your ability to concentrate on tasks requiring coordination is distinctly impaired, especially for driving or operating machinery.

Stupor .15–.30 BAC	=	7–9 drinks/hour or 9–10 drinks/2 hours or 11–13 drinks/3 hours

At this consumption level you become extremely groggy and only semi-alert. This is enough alcohol to shut down your brain alertness centers and cause you to fall asleep or pass out.

Coma .30–.40 BAC	=	10–12 drinks/hour or 13 drinks/2 hours or 14 drinks/3 hours

This quantity of alcohol reduces the amount of oxygen reaching your brain and destroys brain cells at dangerous levels. Unless you have oxygen administered, permanent brain damage may occur.

Death .40–.50 BAC	=	12–15 drinks/hour or 16 drinks/2 hours or 17 drinks/3 hours

Source: *Using Alcohol Responsibly,* Drug Information Center (Eugene, OR: University of Oregon, 1985), p. 5.

glass of wine or a shot of liquor. The effects are the same no matter which one you are drinking. Most people arrested for drunk driving have been drinking beer.

3) *Myth:* I can control the effects that alcohol has on my vision, coordination, and concentration because my willpower is stronger than the alcohol.

Fact: Alcohol is a drug with a chemical composition similar to ether, **Valium**, and other prescription sedatives. Saying that you can resist the effects of alcohol is the same as saying you can resist the effects of Valium. The effects of both are **physiological** and will occur regardless of willpower.

COUNTERMEASURES

Since the 1980s, society has responded to the drinking and driving problem in a number of ways. Groups such as Mothers Against Drunk Driving (MADD), Students Against Driving Drunk (SADD), and Remove Intoxicated Drivers (RID) have brought the problem to the attention of the public and government officials. These groups have lobbied for stronger drunk-driving legislation and stricter enforcement of existing laws.

One of these suggested changes is to lower the legal limit for

Valium: Trademark name for a commonly prescribed brand of diazepam; a mild, psychologically addictive tranquilizer used to relieve anxiety.

Physiological: Related to or a part of the normal, biological functioning of the body.

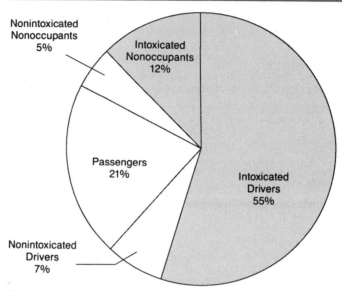

FIGURE 2.3
Traffic Fatalities in Accidents Involving Alcohol

Source: U.S. Department of Transportation, *1989 Traffic Fatality Facts*, p. 2.

Of the 17,850 individuals killed in drunk driving crashes in 1989, 67 percent were themselves intoxicated. The remaining 33 percent were passengers or nonintoxicated drivers or nonintoxicated nonoccupants.

Blood alcohol content (BAC): The percentage of alcohol found in the bloodstream; used to determine levels of intoxication.

Driving While Intoxicated (DWI): Operating a motor vehicle while under the influence of alcohol or other intoxicating drugs.

Diversion programs: Programs designed to "divert" offenders from the normal criminal justice system into educational or therapeutic treatment.

blood alcohol content (BAC) while driving. Most states currently have legal limits of .08 or .10 percent. Proponents suggest that .05 percent would be a more appropriate level, removing a large number of impaired drivers from the highway.

One approach already employed in a number of states involves the establishment of programs to evaluate and treat individuals arrested for **Driving While Intoxicated (DWI)**. Known as **diversion programs** because they "divert" offenders from the normal criminal justice system, these programs seek to classify offenders as social drinkers, beginning problem drinkers, or alcoholics, and provide them with appropriate educational or therapeutic treatment. The goal of these programs is to help offenders overcome their alcohol problems so that they will be less likely to drink and drive in the future.

(continued on p. 36)

The problem: how to cut down on drunk driving, which was killing about 28,000 Americans every year.

Candy Lightner had a horrible reason for wanting to achieve that goal. On May 3, 1980, her 13-year-old daughter Cari was walking to a church carnival in Fair Oaks, Calif., when a car swerved out of control and killed her. Police arrested a 46-year-old cannery worker named Clarence Busch and found that

Candy Lightner's Crusade

he had a long record of arrests for intoxication. Less than a week earlier, he had been bailed out on a hit-and-run drunk-driving charge. A policeman told Lightner that Busch was unlikely to spend any time behind bars for killing her daughter: drunk driving was just one of those things.

Lightner, then 33, a divorced real estate agent with two other children, heard that judgment as she was on her way to a dinner with friends on the eve of her daughter's funeral. She was still furious when she joined them in a cocktail lounge as they waited for a table. It was there, of all places, that she decided to do something. "I remember sitting in the bar with all these people and saying out loud, 'I'm going to start an organization.' Just like that. There was this big moment of silence, and then my girlfriend pipes up and says, 'And we can call it Mothers Against Drunk Drivers.' I didn't have a plan, a goal, nothing. All I knew was that I was going to start an organization, and I was determined to make it work."

She went to see California Governor Jerry Brown to persuade him to appoint a task force to deal with drunk driving. Brown declined to receive her. She went to his office every day, talking to anyone who would listen. After newspapers publicized Lightner's crusade, Brown finally told her that he was appointing the task force and that she would be a member. "I just started crying right there in his office," Lightner says.

Once launched, Mothers Against Drunk Driving (MADD) proved a virtually irresistible force. Now headquartered near Dallas, where Lightner moved, MADD has 320 chapters nationwide and 600,000 volunteers and donors. In response to Lightner's efforts, California passed a tough new law in 1981 that imposes minimum fines of $375 and mandatory imprisonment of up to four years for repeat offenders. By now all 50 states have tightened their drunk-driving laws. And Lightner keeps making speeches, lobbying legislators and generally creating waves. [In] July [1984] she stood beside President Ronald Reagan as he signed a new law reducing federal highway grants to any state that fails to raise the drinking age to 21. Her next goals: an indemnity fund for victims, a bill of rights for victims, automatic imprisonment for repeat offenders. (Clarence Busch did finally serve 21 months in jail for the death of Cari Lightner.)

FIGURE 2.4

Campaigns Against Drunk Driving

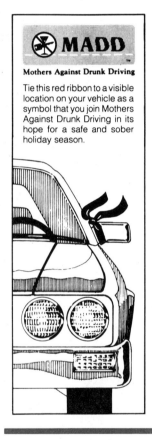

Grass-roots organizations such as Mothers Against Drunk Driving (MADD) have increased the public's awareness of the problems of driving drunk.

Did You Know That . . .

C ommunity residents con-
cerned about dangerous
streets or intersections can ask
their local traffic-safety professionals for pothole repairs, new
signs, lower speed limits, or other
changes.

"I believe that for every problem there is a solution," Lightner
says. "We are changing the way people think about drinking and
driving. But more than that, we have caused people to change their
behavior, and that is saving lives. I believe in the rights of victims. And I
do feel that if you believe in something badly enough, you can make a
difference."

Source: Candy Lightner, "You Can Make a Difference," *Time* (7 January 1985), p. 41.

Public information and targeted education programs are
another approach. Youth traffic safety programs, such as Oregon
Student Safety on the Move (OSSOM), use peer education along
with other activities to help students modify their attitudes about
drinking and driving behavior. These programs aim to teach
students the dangers of drunk driving.

According to the Department of Transportation, there is
evidence to suggest that the communities with the best records of
reducing youthful drinking and driving are those that have
employed a comprehensive community education approach. This
approach involves students, parents, schools, businesses, courts,
and police working together to change the norms of youths'
behavior. The community can promote alcohol-free parties as well
as constructive alternative activities, such as hayrides,
sleighrides, barbecues, bowl-a-thons, ski trips, and canoe trips.

SPEEDING

Drunk driving is one major cause of automobile accidents. Speeding, or driving too fast for road conditions, is another. Speeding
often occurs when the driver is drunk, but other factors also play
a role. Each state keeps its own statistics on speeding, but
because there are no national figures, it is not possible to make
generalizations about speeding that hold for the entire country.
Let us look at Michigan's speeding statistics as an example of a
nationwide problem.

Experts at the Michigan AAA define speeding as "overdriv-
ing the roadway"—in other words, driving too fast for the type of
road or the weather conditions at a given time. Driving a car at a
speed that is safe on an expressway can be dangerous on a two-
lane open-access highway (a roadway with intersecting streets).
According to the AAA, about 90 percent of all Michigan's fatal
accidents occur on this type of road. [5]

(continued on p. 40)

Driving Like the Pros

Driving an automobile, or even riding in one, may be the most dangerous thing you do. At some time in their lives, according to the National Traffic Safety Institute, half of all Americans will be involved in a serious car crash, or will have an immediate family member involved in one. [Safety advocates cite] seat belts, airbags, safer cars, and, of course, sobriety as prime elements in safety. Still, driving skills are an equally important element. You can learn to drive defensively: to avoid putting yourself in a dangerous situation, and to react intelligently in a crisis, should one develop. The box below lists organizations that offer defensive-driving courses. Your insurance agency, police department, or motor vehicle bureau may have additional information.

Think of it this way: the safest driver of all may well be the professional racer. Though he's going 200 mph, he's wearing several seat belts, the chassis in his vehicle is a case of steel tubing, and most important, he's trained to react to danger up ahead. We can't all be racing drivers; yet we could be better drivers than we are. If you've never had a real driving course, and especially if your reaction time isn't as fast as it used to be, defensive-driving training is worth considering. There are other potential benefits, too, besides being a safer driver: most localities will remove citations for moving violations, if any, from your permanent driving record when you complete a course. Most insurance companies offer graduates, particularly those over 55, a break in premiums.

See how you fare on this quiz. (Some questions have more than one correct answer.)

1. The safest way to brake is
   a. as fast as possible.
   b. as far in advance as possible.
2. In moderate town traffic, with another car at a safe distance in front of you, you're being tailgated. What do you do?
   a. Tap the brakes and start to slow down—gradually, keeping an eye on the rearview mirror.
   b. Increase your speed to the allowable limit.
   c. Try to pass the car in front of you.
   d. Pull over to the right.
3. You're heading toward a green light at an intersection. A pedestrian (not in the crosswalk and walking against the light) steps off the curb and starts across without looking. Your first move is to
   a. sound the horn but don't give in. A little scare will do him good.
   b. change lanes to avoid him.
   c. begin braking, anticipating a full stop if necessary, and sound the horn.
4. Preparing to change lanes on a multilane highway, which of the following should you do?
   a. Check your rearview mirror.
   b. Check your side mirror.
   c. Take your eyes off the road momentarily and glance at the lane you're planning to move into.
   d. Turn on your directional signal.
   e. Be aware of what traffic in front of you is doing.
5. You've swerved to the right to avoid a collision on a two-way highway, and your right wheels drop off the pavement and are riding on the shoulder. To get back on the road you
   a. accelerate, cutting the wheel to the left.
   b. don't brake, but take your foot off the accelerator. Hold the wheel steady. When the car slows, check the traffic and steer back onto the pavement.
   c. brake sharply and try to pull off the road altogether. When you've got the car under control, pull onto the road again.
6. On a two-way highway, in what's clearly marked as a no-pass zone with limited visibility, a car pulls out to pass you, and you wonder if he's going to make it. Your best move is to
   a. speed up, hoping he'll duck behind you.
   b. ignore him—it's his problem.

c. reduce your speed so he can get around you faster.

7. The most important factor in defensive driving is
   a. quick reflexes.
   b. anticipating trouble.
   c. skill at vehicle handling.
   d. strict observation of the law.

8. You're most likely to go into a skid
   a. in a steady downpour.
   b. in the first few minutes of a light rain.

9. Which of the following road conditions up ahead should tell you to reduce your speed?
   a. A deep pothole.
   b. Leaves on the pavement.
   c. Any bridge, when the temperature is just above freezing.

10. Your car is skidding (see diagram). What's the safest reaction?
   a. Turn the wheel to the right.
   b. Turn the wheel to the left.
   c. Brake as hard as possible and avoid turning the wheel until you've stopped the car.

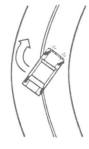

11. In two-way highway traffic, an oncoming car suddenly pulls into your lane. What action do you take?
   a. Brake hard and sound your horn.
   b. Move quickly into the left lane.
   c. Blow your horn, and head to the shoulder.

12. The best position for your hands on the steering wheel is
   a. at "10" and "2" o'clock position.
   b. at "8" and "4" o'clock.
   c. wherever you're most comfortable.
   d. at "9" and "3" o'clock.

13. True or false: Underinflated tires are safer, particularly in hot weather.

14. You realize you're heading into a curve too fast. Therefore you should
   a. brake sharply.
   b. brake gradually.

c. avoid braking but take your foot off the accelerator.

ANSWERS

1. (b) A basic principle of defensive driving is never to get into a situation that calls for slamming on the brakes. This can throw you into a skid and injure you and your passengers. Good braking technique: pump the brakes, reapplying as you come to a full stop. However, according to Professor Donald Smith, Highway Traffic Safety Program, Michigan State University, if you are forced to brake fast and have disc brakes, "threshold" braking is the best technique: push the brake just short of locking and hold it there.

2. (a) and **(d)**, depending on circumstances. If the tailgater is daydreaming, tapping your brakes (and activating the brake lights) should wake him up. If he's being aggressive, you've politely signaled him to let up. If he doesn't stop tailgating, pull over as soon as you can and let him pass.

3. (c) Always yield the right of way to a pedestrian, even when he's in the wrong. Let him know you're there. A diversionary swerve could put you in the path of an oncoming car. Also, the pedestrian might dart into your pathway.

4. (all) All steps are essential, but some people forget (c). You always have a blind spot (about a car length behind you on either side) and may not be able to see an overtaking vehicle in either mirror. Always glance over your shoulder before making your move. The signal light (turned on several seconds in advance) will help protect you as well.

5. (b) Braking hard or jerking the wheel can cause you to skid into oncoming traffic. Don't brake but do reduce your speed and stay on a steady course. Then, after checking traffic, make a sharp quarter turn to the left to put yourself back on the road, then straighten out.

6. (c) Passing is always a cooperative venture. If this reckless driver has a head-on collision, you might be hurt, too.

7. (b) Obeying the law and vehicle-handling skills are all important. But anticipating trouble up ahead, and acting to prevent it, can make the speed of your reflexes far less important and thus may prevent many collisions.

8. (b) A little water plus the oil and dirt on the road form a slick film. A heavy rain will wash it clean. Be extra careful during the first half hour of a rainfall.

9. (all) The pothole may only jar you, but it could damage your car or even cause you to lose control. Leaves can send you into a skid. And even though there's no ice on the road, a bridge is about 6°F colder than a highway and may be hazardous when the road is not.

10. (b) Turn the wheel straight down your lane. That is, if your rear wheels are skidding left, as in the diagram, turn with the skid—that is, to the left. Don't brake, as this increases skidding.

11. (c) Don't move left, which could put you in someone else's pathway. Always move right when heading off the road.

12. (d) and some expert drivers recommend that you hook your thumbs lightly over the horizontal spokes. This gives you a feel for the front tires and is a good way to get a quick grip if you strike a pothole.

13. False. An underinflated tire is more likely to skid, whether in hot weather or on wet or icy pavement. Because underinflation allows a tire to "flap" slightly and thus to create more heat, it's also likelier to blow out. Even for desert driving, keep tires at the recommended maximum air pressure, and check them weekly. The number should be printed on the side of the tires; or check the instruction manual if the car still has its original tires.

14. (b) Take your foot off the accelerator, and brake before you get into the curve, but gradually release brakes as you get into it. Once you're rounding the curve, accelerate. This will help you steer safely around it and onto the straightaway.

Better brakes down the road

The onboard automotive computer may one day contribute substantially to highway safety. One application that's already in limited use is the antilock brake. Activated by a sensor attached to each car wheel, these brakes detect potential skids and react accordingly, pulsing the brake power and bringing the vehicle to a faster, safer stop than conventional brakes, especially in hazardous road conditions such as ice and snow. The European Economic Community now requires antilock brakes on trucks and buses, but the U.S., unfortunately, does not. Antilock brakes are now standard equipment on some cars in the luxury category and optional on some others (at a cost of about $1,000). By the year 2000, antilock brakes will probably be standard on all passenger cars, at much lower cost.

Driving schools

For information about defensive-driving courses in your area, write or telephone:

American Association of Retired Persons, Attention: 55 Alive, 1909 K Street NW, Washington, DC 20049; 202-662-4863.

National Traffic Safety Institute, 275 North 4th Street, San Jose, CA 95112; 800-732-2233 (west of the Mississippi), 800-334-1441 (elsewhere).

National Safety Council, 444 North Michigan Avenue, Chicago, IL 60611 (include self-addressed stamped envelope).

The two-second rule

To be sure you're following at a safe distance, pick out some definite marker (a driveway, a bridge abutment, a sign) on the road ahead, and when the car in front of you passes it, start counting seconds, "one thousand and one, one thousand and two." Two seconds should elapse before your own car reaches the marker. In bad weather, when it's harder to stop, make it four seconds. That gives you a safety cushion of space.

Source: *University of California Berkeley Wellness Letter,* October 1989, pp. 4–5.

Did You Know That . . .

Roads are most hazardous for cyclists in the first 30 minutes of a rainstorm, when slicks consisting of motor vehicle oils and gasoline have spread but not yet been washed away.

MOTORCYCLE ACCIDENTS

Automobile driving has its hazards, but it is a much safer mode of transportation than motorcycle driving. In 1989 the death rate for automobile drivers and passengers was approximately 2.25 per 100,000,000 miles driven. [6] For motorcycle riders, the rate was 29 deaths per 100,000,000 miles driven. [7] In other words, in 1989 motorcyclists were more than 12 times as likely to die as were car drivers.

FIGURE 2.5
Safe Motorcycling

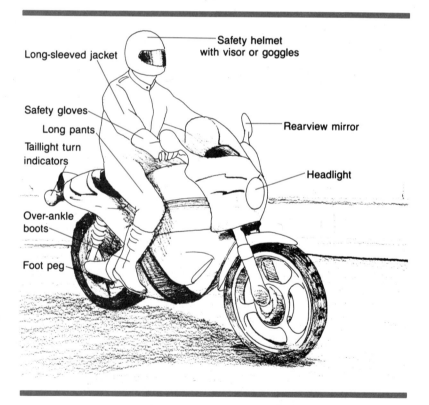

A safety helmet with a visor, gloves, heavy shoes or boots, and leather or other heavy clothing can help protect the motorcyclist from serious injury. Proper use of turn signals, headlight, taillight, and rearview mirrors can help the rider avoid an accident.

Why is there such a huge difference? A study by H. H. Hurt at the Traffic Safety Center of the University of Southern California shed some light on some of the reasons.

Surprisingly, almost 50 percent of the motorcycle accidents Hurt studied occurred when a car or truck ran into the motorcycle, rather than the other way around. [8] This occurred most often at an intersection, where an automobile turned into the path of the oncoming motorcycle. Many car drivers involved in such accidents explained their role by noting that, accustomed to looking for larger vehicles, they just overlooked the oncoming motorcycle. In other cases, the driver of the car was intoxicated at the time of the collision.

Hurt's study did not hold motorcycle drivers blameless, however. The study implicated motorcyclists in about 45 percent of the accidents. [9] In these cases, alcohol intoxication was often the problem. Perhaps the tendency of some motorcyclists to take advantage of the small size of motorcyles to weave in and out of traffic, ignoring normal passing laws, was also a factor. In addition, it was found that the least experienced and least trained motorcyclists were more likely to be involved in fatalities. Ninety-two percent of the riders were self-taught or taught by family members. Fifty percent had fewer than 5 months' experience on the motorcycle they were riding and fewer than 3 years' overall riding experience. [10]

Only about 5 percent of the accidents were caused by equipment or roadway defects. The most common of these were flat tires and failed brakes.

PEDESTRIAN ACCIDENTS

Eighteen percent of motor vehicle accidents in this country each year involve pedestrians. More than half of these occur when pedestrians enter or cross the streets. Studies show that individuals under the age of 4 and over the age of 75 have the highest pedestrian fatality rates. [11]

Many parents overestimate the abilities of their children as pedestrians. A number of experts agree that children under the age of 10 cannot safely cope with traffic. Many fail to see or hear motor vehicles approaching from the side or rear. Younger children cannot comprehend signs and signals and frequently misinterpret them. Many children cannot predict the speed of motor vehicles or understand how long it takes them to stop. Youngsters do not realize that a motor vehicle traveling at 40 mph requires

Think you know how to walk? Don't laugh; the question isn't as silly as it seems.

With an ever-increasing consciousness about health and wellness, more people than ever are making a brisk walk an important part of their daily routine. That's fine, but there is a downside to walking, if you don't take a few simple precautions.

It's Time to Learn How to Walk—Defensively

Each year, more than 7,000 pedestrians are killed by motor vehicles, and another 80,000 or so are injured. Experts maintain pedestrian-vehicle accidents are usually the fault of the pedestrian. . . .

Surprisingly, these accidents don't happen at night; most victims are injured or killed between 3 and 5 p.m., in fair, warm weather. And that is just the kind of weather in which most people like to take their walks.

Urban walkers account for about 60 percent of all fatalities, and those over age 65 are most prone. You should take heed of the following safety tips, to become a good, defensive walker and minimize your risk of meeting a motor vehicle by accident:

- On a "walk" or green light, wait and look. Just because you have the right to cross the street doesn't mean a car isn't coming, running the light, etc.
- Make eye contact with the motorist before crossing.
- Don't step blindly from a parked car.
- Be especially alert when crossing in a right-hand-turn lane.
- Avoid jaywalking; always use a crosswalk.
- Always walk facing traffic. If you're a recreational walker, always carry a flashlight at night and wear reflective clothing, especially if you walk in areas of steady or high traffic.
- Always expect the unexpected. Be alert for swerving cars, speeders, and other types of erratic drivers.

Source: *Saint Raphael's Better Health*, November/December 1989, p. 10.

well over 100 feet to come to a full stop. It cannot stop on a dime in the way that they or their tricycles can.

Children are not the only age group at risk as pedestrians. The elderly account for approximately one-fourth of all pedestrian deaths. Among the reasons for this are that some elderly people suffer hearing and vision impairments that affect their depth perception. In addition, the limited mobility and physical

FIGURE 2.6
Traffic Signals for Bicyclists

Left turns

Look over your left shoulder to scan
traffic, signal when clear, and then
take the left lane when safe. Signal in-
tention to turn left by extending left
hand horizontally.

Right turns

Extend right hand horizontally.

Slowing or stopping

Extend left hand downward.

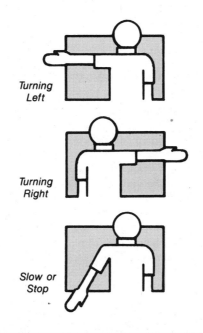

*Turning
Left*

*Turning
Right*

*Slow or
Stop*

Bicyclists are required to obey all regulatory signs and signals on the road and have
all duties and rights of motorists. A bell or horn is required to alert others of a bicycle
approaching.

frailty of some elderly people make it more difficult for them to
move quickly out of the way of traffic.

The young and the old are not the only groups who are
vulnerable to roadside accidents. Joggers, skateboarders, and
roller skaters are a relatively new pedestrian hazard. Because
joggers are constantly moving, drivers may have problems detect-
ing how far they are from the vehicle. Many joggers are very
aggressive and tend not to stop at intersections, challenging the
right-of-way of the motor vehicle. Jogging is much more dangerous at night when the poor visibility of both runners and
drivers leads to more accidents. Joggers who run at night *must*
wear reflective clothing. In addition, they should avoid wearing

(continued on p. 45)

Cycling is one of the best forms of exercise around: it gives the heart and circulatory system an aerobic workout; it puts little stress on joints; it can burn between 400 and 700 calories per hour; if you own a bike, cycling is free; and it can be done just about anywhere.

But there are some steps you can take to improve cycling safety and enjoyment:

17 Tips for the Savvy Cyclist

Braking

- Brake with your hands at the end of the levers. This will allow you to exert optimal pressure.
- Don't brake abruptly during the first minutes of a rainstorm, when roads are especially slippery.
- On long, steep downhills, as well as in wet weather, it is safest to "feather brake"—that is, tap the brakes, applying intermittent pressure.
- For a quick stop, as you press the brakes firmly, slide your buttocks to the very back of the saddle. This will keep the rear of the bike down so that you don't flip over the handlebars.
- Don't jam on the brakes, however, or you may lose control of the bike. The front brake (the left lever) has the power to stop you more quickly than the back (the right lever), but when squeezed too hard it can throw you over the handlebars. The back brake, with strong pressure, may cause the bicycle to skid.

The right stuff

- Always wear a helmet. This is the most important precaution a cyclist can take. Of the nation's 1,000 annual cycling deaths, head injuries account for about 85% of them.
- When cycling at night or whenever visibility is poor, wear brightly colored, reflective clothing, and use your headlight. In fact, wearing bright colors is a good idea at any time.
- Don't wear headphones. They can block out most of the street sounds you need to hear in order to ride defensively. Wearing headphones while cycling is a misdemeanor in some municipalities.
- Don't wear a heavy backpack. It can throw you off balance. Carry packages only in baskets, handlebar or seat bags, or panniers (side pouches made especially for bicycles).

Good road sense

- Use hand signals. This will allow the drivers of the cars around you to anticipate your actions.
- Learn to change gears without taking your eyes off the road so that you won't swerve into traffic.
- Watch out for storm drains, cattle guards (for country riders), and

railroad tracks. They're all slippery when wet. And if you don't cross them at a right angle, your front tire may get caught, causing you to be thrown off your bike.
* Don't ride side by side with another cyclist in traffic. Use bike lanes, when available.

Make it easy

* Don't ride in the racing "drop" position (with your hands on the curved part of the handlebars) for any extended period of time. Though this position does make you a bit more aerodynamic and thus makes your pedaling more efficient, it may cramp your hands, shoulders, and neck. Instead, ride with your hands over the tops of the handlebars and switch hand positions frequently.
* After a long uphill, don't coast downhill without pedaling. As you climb up the hill, lactic acid builds up in your muscles and can contribute to muscle soreness; by pedaling lightly but constantly while coasting downhill (even if there's little resistance), you can help remove the lactic acid.
* Wear shoes with rigid soles. These allow for more efficient pedaling, since they usually transmit more power to the pedals.
* Keep your arms relaxed, and don't lock your elbows. This technique helps you absorb bumps from the road better. Also, when you see bumps ahead in the road, raise your buttocks slightly off the seat, keeping your knees bent—this will prevent you from bouncing painfully on the seat.

Source: *University of California Berkeley Wellness Letter,* June 1990, p. 6.

tape players or radios with headsets, which can make it impossible to hear such sounds as sirens, horns, or vehicle engines.

In general, joggers should observe the following safety suggestions:

1. If at all possible, do not jog in areas of heavy vehicle traffic. If jogging paths or trails are available, use them. It is best to avoid running on streets altogether, but if you must run on a roadway, choose one with a wide shoulder.

2. Always jog facing traffic.

3. Nighttime jogging can be very dangerous. If you must run after dark, wear a reflective vest or other bright garment that can be seen clearly by drivers.

(continued on p. 47)

Cycling Safely in Traffic

If you're a cyclist who's been rattled by your initial experiences with motor traffic, this might sound crazy: The solution is to make life easier for drivers. It's true because it's in our self-interest to make the road a safer, more pleasant place. Even though you may fantasize about getting even with rude or aggressive drivers, it seldom helps. A better policy is to minimize the chance for conflict in the first place.

Here are nine easy ways to share the road peacefully and, above all, keep friendly drivers friendly. These tips are particularly effective for cyclists who are still developing their confidence, fitness, and bike-handling ability.

1. Keep right—This most basic rule of sharing the road is the one that cyclists are most casual about. If there's a wide, clean shoulder, use it. Barring potholes, storm grates, parked cars, glass, gravel, and other hazards, most of the time it's easier (and safer) to stay to the right. One thing that always irritates motorists is a cyclist riding in the middle of the road for no apparent reason.

2. Use common sense about riding two or more abreast—Sure, it's enjoyable to ride side by side with a companion and carry on a conversation. But road and traffic conditions may be such that vehicles back up behind and then pass dangerously when they could otherwise slip safely by. It's usually best to restrict side-by-side riding to quiet, secondary roads.

3. Don't force vehicles to repass you needlessly—You're riding along a narrow, busy road and motorists are having trouble getting by. There are a dozen cars waiting at the next red light, all of which have already patiently overtaken you. Do you maintain your place in line, or do you zip past everyone on the right so you'll get the jump when the light changes? If you do the latter, you might gain 50 feet and save a few seconds, but you'll also probably create 12 anti-bicyclists when they get caught behind you again.

Admittedly, the scenario becomes trickier if, by hanging back, you miss the light. There are two tactful ways around this: One is to only move up in line far enough to just make the light. The other is to ride to the light, but move out slowly and slightly to the right when it turns green, letting the cars through the intersection first. One other courtesy at traffic lights: Avoid blocking drivers who want to turn right on red.

4. Ride predictably—Maintain a straight line when you're cruising, and use hand signals when turning or changing lanes.

If you ride erratically, it's difficult for drivers to know when to pass. They may let several relatively safe opportunities go by before becoming exasperated and taking a dangerous chance.

Hand signals are a courtesy and an important part of safe cycling. Motorists feel more comfortable dealing with cyclists who communicate their intentions. More important, drivers tend to show them more respect. Use the same hand signals that motorists use, except for a right turn, which is indicated by pointing with your right arm.

5. Avoid busy roads—It's surprising how often you see cyclists on a busy highway, ruffling the delicate feathers of already edgy commuters. An alternate route doesn't have to be a residential street with stop signs every block or a glass-littered, jogger-strewn bike path. Examine a detailed map of your area and you'll probably find a relatively quiet road that takes you where you want to go.

6. Make yourself visible—In conditions where motorists might not readily see you (an overcast day, for example), it's a courtesy and plain good sense to wear brightly colored clothes. Drivers will never blame themselves when they almost pull into your path after a too-casual look. Unfair, yes; but you can greatly enhance your safety by dressing to be seen.

At night, it's a different story. Drivers who encounter dark-clothed cyclists riding without lights and reflectors are right to consider them menaces.

7. Be careful about "provocative" actions—At a red light, even friendly drivers are likely to be irritated by a cyclist riding in circles in front of them. Many view it as a challenge to their right-of-way, even when none is intended. Similarly, if you lean on a vehicle at a stoplight, be aware that most drivers consider their cars extensions of themselves. You wouldn't want someone leaning on your bike, would you?

Even minor gestures can be taken the wrong way by motorists. Unfortunately, some have had ill experiences with cyclists, so their fuses are already lit. Be careful with hand motions of any type, and save all one-finger salutes for the stadium to signify that your favorite team is No. 1.

8. Return the favor—Cyclists come to appreciate little unexpected courtesies from motorists. For instance, we all nod a thank you to the driver who has the right-of-way but waves us through anyway. Try returning the favor. You might, for example, motion a driver to make his turn in front of you if you'll be slow getting under way. Who knows? That driver might look a bit more favorably on the next cyclist down the road.

9. Obey traffic laws—Probably nothing irritates motorists more than watching a cyclist blithely sail through a stop sign or light with barely a reduction in speed. "Who does that guy think he is?" is the usual reaction, and all cyclists suffer by association. If we want to be treated with courtesy and respect by motorists, acting as if we're superior won't make it happen. And legally, we're bound by the same laws as drivers in all states. If you run a light or commit any other traffic offense you can be fined, so ride your bike as you'd drive your car.

RULES OF THE ROAD

These are the keys to increasing your safety in the midst of motor vehicles.

- Always ride on the right. Go with the flow of traffic, never against it.
- Be predictable. Maintain a straight line, change direction without swerving, and use hand signals when turning.
- Obey all traffic laws. If you want to be safe in traffic you have to act like traffic.
- Pay attention. Use your eyes and ears as warning devices, alerting you to potential hazards in time to take action.
- Assert yourself. Don't let vehicles creep by and force you into parked cars or the curb. You have a legal right to the lane, so take as much as you need for safety.
- Ride defensively. Expect a car to pull out from the side street or turn left in front of you. If you anticipate the worst it will rarely happen.
- Be visible. Wear bright colors and put reflectors and reflective tape on your bicycle.
- Shout. It's the quickest, most effective way to let a motorist know that he or she is putting you in danger, or to alert an inattentive pedestrian that you are approaching.

Source: The editors of *Bicycling* magazine (Emmaus, PA, 1990).

4. At intersections, make sure drivers see you before crossing. Make eye contact with them.

5. Be aware of what is going on around you. It is a common sight to see runners listening to music while jogging, a dangerous practice that can lull them into forgetting about safety.

6. Do not challenge cars or agitate drivers; you are no match for a 3,000-pound car.

Did You Know That . . .

To choose a bike sized correctly for a child, make sure he or she can keep both feet on the ground while straddling the top horizontal bar.

BICYCLE SAFETY

Bicycle riding has become increasingly popular in the United States. Unfortunately, the recent resurgence in the sport has led to a higher prevalence of bicycle-related fatalities and injuries.

A look at bicycle accident statistics provides some insight into the causes of accidents. Not surprisingly, 90 percent of bicycle fatalities are caused by collisions with automobiles. Fifty percent of such collisions occur in the intersections of sidewalks, driveways, and streets. The most common errors made by bicycle riders that result in accidents are failure to signal a turn or lane change properly and failure to ride in the proper lane. Males, possibly because of greater risk-taking behavior, are twice as likely to be involved in a bicycle accident. [12]

As we have seen, traffic safety is a complex problem that involves the interaction of drivers, motor vehicles, motorcycles, bicycles, pedestrians, and **environmental factors**. Motor vehicle operators, bicyclists, and pedestrians can take simple steps that greatly reduce their risk of accidental death or injury. Avoiding alcohol use when driving and following the other safety precautions listed in this chapter can take much of the life-or-death gamble out of venturing onto our streets and highways. W

Environmental factors:
Factors such as weather and road hazards external to the individuals, and any objects or devices immediately involved in an accident.

Accidents in the Home

3

IT MAY BE TRUE that your home is your castle, but without proper precautions, it can be a dangerous one. Injuries occur more often from accidents at home than anywhere else. The number of deaths from home accidents is second only to deaths in automobile mishaps, and the yearly economic cost of home accidents is close to $17 billion. The most vulnerable family members—elders and the very young—suffer the majority of these accidents.

FALLS

Most fatal home accidents are caused by falls. These most often afflict older adults: of the 12,400 deaths from falls in 1989, 9,350 involved persons over the age of 65. [1]

There are 2 reasons why falls take such a large toll among older adults. First, the elderly are more likely to fall. The decline in vision, hearing, and balance that often accompanies the aging process can greatly reduce the ability to identify and avoid obstacles or to maintain balance when an obstacle cannot be avoided. In addition, many older people take medications that can cause dizziness or disorientation when taken in the wrong dosage, mixed with other prescriptions, or taken with alcohol.

The second reason so many of the elderly are injured or killed in falls is that they are more vulnerable. Bone mass tends to diminish with age, which leaves older people more susceptible to fractures than younger people. Although children under 5 also suffer many falls, they have stronger bones and greater flexibility than older people and are less likely to suffer serious injury. The older person's body is also less able to heal itself, which means that fractures can be debilitating or even fatal.

Wise Precautions

Most falls occur on stairways, in bathrooms, or in bedrooms. Giving some attention to these areas can go a long way toward protecting an older family member. Use nonskid floor coverings, sturdy handrails, and proper lighting on stairways. Keep the

(continued on p. 52)

Preventing Falls

As a Minnesota grandmother stepped into her bathtub, the bathmat scooted from under her feet and she fell hard, breaking her hip.

In Chicago, a 4-year-old playing fireman with his sister fell three stories from a fire escape to his death on the pavement below.

I was luckier, if not wiser. Carrying a big load of laundry that obscured my view, I slipped on a boxing glove left lying on the steps. By some miracle, the fall did not break my back, but I got a severe bruise and it was months before I could sit or run with comfort.

More often than not, falls are preventable. Falls are the second leading cause of accidental death, after motor vehicle accidents; among the elderly, falls rank first. Not only are older people more likely to have health problems that increase their likelihood of falling, they are also more susceptible to devastating injuries, such as hip fractures, because their bones are often weakened by osteoporosis.

In 1985, 6,300 people died in falls at home, half of all home-related deaths, and 4,900 of the victims were 65 or older. Falls account for two-thirds of deaths at home among people aged 75 and older.

Among older people who survive a fall, two-thirds are likely to fall again within six months. Twenty percent of elderly people living at home fall in a given year, and the incidence of falls at home is twice that of ambulatory elderly people living in institutions. Of the 210,000 hip fractures among Americans each year, 90 percent result from falls.

In cities, falls from apartment windows, rooftops and fire escapes continue to be a serious problem, even in a city like New York, which requires guards on windows in apartments where children under 10 live.

A study published in June 1986 by Dr. Sylvia M. Ramos and Dr. Harry M. Delany reported that in a five-year period 203 victims of falls from heights were brought to one hospital in the Bronx. Of these, 76 percent suffered severe injuries, including permanent brain damage, and 28 percent died. Most of the falls were deemed accidental.

In many cases, falls are accidents that were waiting to happen. If the possibility of a fall had been considered in advance, at least two-thirds could easily have been avoided.

The Minnesota grandmother, for example, who is 77, knew the bathmat was unreliable: she had slipped on it twice before, luckily escaping injury. Yet she neglected to replace it with something safer, such as nonskid strips. Nor had she handrails to help her get into and out of the tub.

After six months in a nursing home she returned home to find that her family and friends had, among other things, installed safety rails in the bathroom, rubber treads and a sturdy new bannister on the stairs and handy new light switches, and had tacked down electrical cords throughout the house. She made further improvements, moving furniture to widen the paths between rooms.

Causes

Physical, psychological and environmental factors can increase the chances of falling, especially for older people. As people age their vision may become impaired, and if areas are not well-lighted they may fail to see obstacles or steps in time. Gait or balance may become unsteady, perhaps due to an illness like Parkinson's disease or arthritis.

Older people are also more likely to get dizzy when standing up after lying down or when bending over, because blood pressure to the head does not rise fast enough. This is a common problem, for example, among patients receiving drug therapy for high blood pressure.

Other medications, such as tranquilizers, antidepressants and antianxiety drugs, can lead to dizziness and falls. The elderly are also more sensitive to the disorienting effects of alcohol. Sometimes heart disease or disorders that affect mental functions increase the risk of falling.

Elderly people may also resist asking others for help and instead attempt activities—climbing to reach a top shelf for instance—that are beyond their physical abilities. In some, depression impairs their awareness of their surroundings.

In the living environment, uneven pavements or steps, slippery floors or rugs, unexpected door thresholds, obtrusive furniture or wires, and inadequate support on stairways increase the chances of an older person falling.

Prevention

The following measures, recommended by, among others, *Drug Therapy,* a magazine for physicians, can help diminish the chances of falling at any age:

- Clean up spills immediately, using soap and rinsing well if the spill was greasy.
- Never place anything on a staircase or at the head or foot of a stairway.
- Be sure stairs are in good repair and steps are evenly spaced. If possible, cover steps with permanently attached nonskid treads and install handrails on both sides of the stairway. Place a strip of glow-in-the-dark tape on the top and bottom steps. For outside steps and walkways, keep a pail of sand, salt or ice-melting compound handy, and keep steps and sidewalks in good repair.
- Stairways and hallways should be well-lighted, with switches at either end. If possible, install switches that are illuminated when in the off position, and use night lights or remote-controlled bedside switches for routes between bedrooms and baths.
- Never carry a load that obscures your vision. If glasses are needed to see nearby objects, always wear them, even to go to the bathroom in the night.
- Use only sturdy step stools or ladders to reach things high up. Never climb on a chair or cabinet, carton or stack of books. Avoid using the top step of a stepladder; if your ladder is too short, get a taller ladder.
- Install carpeting or runners on slippery floors. If loose rugs are used, place them on nonskid pads and tack or tape them to the floor. Wear rubber-soled shoes, especially at home, to reduce the chances of slipping on uncarpeted floors.
- Install safety railings and support handles in the bathroom, especially around the tub and toilet. Affix nonslip strips to the bottom of the tub, or use a mat with section cups that hold firm when they are stepped on. To assure good suction, place the mat in the tub only when the tub is dry.
- Do not let electrical cords hang loose. Gather and tie them to the length needed, or tape or tack them to the wall or the edge of the floor.
- If small children live in the house, install window guards. Screens are not adequate protection. Never leave a small child unattended near an open window or on an upper-story deck or rooftop with a low fence.
- If you often get dizzy or feel faint when you sit up or stand up quickly, try the following: sleep with your head raised, wear elastic stockings, get up slowly after sitting or lying down, sit on the edge of the bed for a minute or so before trying to stand, then stand by the bed briefly before trying to walk. In addition, see your doctor, since a change in medication may be needed.

Source: Jane Brody, "Personal Health," *New York Times* (3 December 1986), p. C4.

Did You Know That . . .

Falls account for approximately 1.4 million visits each year to hospital emergency rooms in the United States.

FIGURE 3.1
Bathroom Safety Features for Older or Disabled People

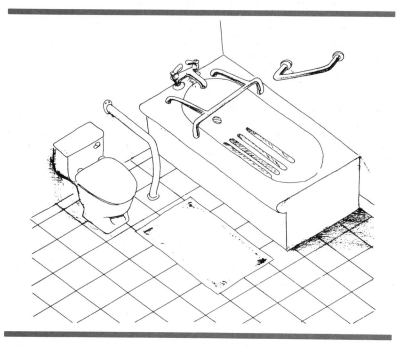

Many falls can be avoided if handrails are installed near the bathtub and toilet, and nonslip mats are used inside and alongside the bathtub.

stairs clear of toys, tools, shoes, and other obstacles. Nonslip surfaces should also be used in tubs and showers; newer tubs are sometimes made with special embossed or textured bottoms. Older tubs can be fitted with nonslip decals or mats. Older adults should have firmly anchored grab rails placed along the sides of the tub to help them enter and exit safely. Installing a night-light is an additional safety measure useful for late-night journeys to the kitchen or bathroom.

POISONINGS

Ingest: To take in by swallowing; to eat.

Whereas older adults are the most vulnerable to falls, the very young are highly susceptible to accidental poisonings. Every year about 2 million Americans inadvertently **ingest** or inhale poi-

FIGURE 3.2
The Home Medicine Cabinet

Approximately 75,000 calls to poison control centers each year are from parents of children who have eaten a household or garden plant.

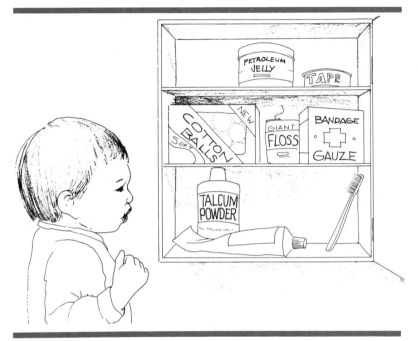

The medicine cabinet may seem the logical place to keep prescription drugs and medications, but not if you have young children at home. It is safer to keep medicines in a locked cabinet out of reach of all children. Store only nontoxic substances in a cabinet that can be opened by children or toddlers.

sonous substances. [2] Although most of these poisonings are nonfatal, every year about 6,000 result in death. [3]

Most fatal poisonings occur in the home and involve common household substances such as medications, insecticides, petroleum products, cleaning agents, garden and lawn products, and fumes. Even plants found around the home can be dangerous. The Oregon Poison Control Center has reported that exposure to plants, including houseplants, lawn and garden plants, and mushrooms, is second only to drug overdoses in generating calls to the Center.

Children are the primary victims of poisonings for a number of reasons. Infants and toddlers explore their surroundings by taste-testing everything, including **toxic substances**. Without

(continued on p. 55)

Toxic substances: Substances that are harmful or poisonous.

As your child's world expands from the playpen to the playroom, home sweet home provides continual adventure. And constant hazard.

Look at your environment from the little one's perspective: What's safe for you can be dangerous for him or her. For example, every year one in 20 children under age 5 is accidentally poisoned by substances found in the home, according to the National Safety Council.

Out of Danger's Reach

To help keep your children away from the frying pan and out of the fire, try these safety pointers:

Children from birth to 6 months are quickly learning to roll over, wiggle and push against things with their feet. Do not leave your baby unattended in high places, such as changing tables, beds and sofas. Put safety gates on all stairways—top and bottom—when your child begins to crawl.

Mattresses should fit snugly inside a child's crib. And no pillows! Infants have little control of their heads and could roll face down and suffocate. Once children can pull themselves up, "crib gyms" become strangulation hazards. Remove them from the crib when the child is unsupervised. Also, lower your water heater temperature to between 120 and 130 degrees Fahrenheit. The lower temperature greatly reduces your child's risk of being scalded by tap water.

Children 7 to 12 months old start to put everything within clutching distance into their mouths, and therefore are particularly susceptible to poisoning and choking. Never leave small objects—such as hard candy, buttons and coins—within reach of your child. Keep all medicines and hazardous materials locked up and out of reach; make sure they have childproof caps. Place your local poison control center's phone number within immediate reach of all your phones and be sure to have a bottle of syrup of ipecac on hand to induce vomiting. (Note: Ipecac should be used only on the instruction of your doctor or poison control center.)

At this age, your child will probably love playing in water. Never leave him or her unattended around water, even for a few seconds. A few inches of water is all it takes to drown a child.

Children 1 to 2 years old will be walking, climbing and riding. These new means of transportation greatly increase early exploration efforts—but also increase the risk of falls. Pad sharp edges of furniture. When cooking, keep your child away from the stove in a secure place such as a highchair or playpen.

Keep small objects that may cause choking, as well as dangerous instruments (knives, scissors, tools), out of sight and out of reach. Kitchen cabinets are magnets for a curious toddler; keep your child out of harm's way by installing child-resistant latches. Store all toxic household products in one cabinet and make sure it's locked.

Children 2 to 4 years old are running and may have mastered tricycles and Big Wheels™ by now. As children increase their ground speed and mayhem potential, stairs and windows become major hazards. To lessen the risks, make sure screens and storm windows are securely in place and that gates are on the stairs.

Other safety tips for children of all ages: Place safety plugs in wall sockets that are not in use. Store hazardous chemicals in their original containers in well-ventilated places. Your yard and houseplants can be hidden threats: Call your poison control center for a list of poisonous plants.

You may want to consider replacing certain household products—especially those containing lye—with non-toxic (and environmentally safe) alternatives. *Drains:* Pour boiling water with ¼ cup baking soda down drains to clear most clogs. *Windows:* Mix 3 tablespoons vinegar with 1 quart warm water for window cleaner. *Ovens:* Use a mixture of baking soda and water; scrub with steel wool. Contact a local environmental group for a list of other alternative cleaning aids.

Source: *Health Action,* Vol. 1, No. 3, March 1991, p. 3.

hesitation they may drink cleaning or lawn products, swallow medications, or chew on household plants.

Older children who have outgrown the taste-testing stage but are still too young to understand the dangers of some products can also be harmed. They may take their parents' medications while playing "grown-up" or "hospital," or they may mix and drink toxic substances as part of other play activities. Some parents try to entice their children to take medicine by calling it candy; in some cases, medications are actually flavored and packaged like candy. These deceptions can lead mischievous children to raid the medicine cabinet looking for a treat.

A very small percentage of children are among those afflicted with a condition called **pica**, which causes an unnatural craving for nonfood substances such as paint chips, dirt, coal, or plaster. For obvious reasons such children are particularly susceptible to poisonings.

Poison Prevention and Treatment
One way to prevent poisonings is to monitor children closely, especially infants and toddlers. Unfortunately, monitoring is not always foolproof. It is impossible to watch a child every moment, and a poisoning can occur in a matter of seconds. A better safeguard is to monitor the poisonous substances themselves.

(continued on p. 59)

Pica: A condition characterized by a craving for normally inedible substances; it is thought to be caused by a hormonal or nutritional deficiency.

Chemical Hazards in the Home

When you think of chemical hazards, you may think of Bhopal or the Love Canal. But these isolated industrial cases represent more immediate problems that affect you daily. Hazardous chemicals are present in virtually every American home—they're in your cleanser, your disinfectants, even the motor oil in your garage.

Hazardous household chemicals can be grouped into four categories:

Reactive products contain unstable compounds that may react with air, water, or other chemicals with dangerous results. One example is calcium hypochlorite, a powder used to disinfect swimming pools, which can react with paint or kerosene to produce explosive and toxic chlorine gas.

Corrosives are strong acids or bases that eat away other substances. Examples include chlorine bleach, a powerful acid, and drain opener, a powerful base. Corrosives can cause severe burns on contact, and their vapors can burn the eyes. They are also poisonous if ingested.

Ignitable products, like gasoline and furniture polish, pose a fire hazard if improperly stored or used.

Toxic products have perhaps the greatest po-

Chemical Hazards in the Home

Product	Possible Hazards	Disposal Suggestions	Precautions and Substitutes
Aerosols	When sprayed, contents are broken into particles small enough to be inhaled. Cans may explode or burn.	Put **only** empty cans in trash. Do not burn. Do not place in trash compactor.	Store in cool place. Propellant may be flammable. Instead: use non-aerosol products.
Drain cleaners	Very corrosive. May be fatal if swallowed. Contact with eyes can cause blindness.	Use up according to label instructions.	Prevention best; keep sink strainers in good condition. Instead: use plunger, plumber's snake, vinegar & baking soda followed by boiling water.
Flea powders, sprays & shampoos	Moderately to very poisonous. *Toxicity 2–4˙*	Use up or save for hazardous waste collection day.	DO NOT USE DOG PRODUCTS ON CATS Vacuum house regularly & thoroughly. Launder pet bedding frequently.
Oven cleaner	Corrosive. Very harmful if swallowed. Irritating vapors. Can cause eye damage. *Toxicity 2–4˙*	Use up according to label instructions or give away. Save for hazardous waste collection day.	Do not use aerosols, which can explode and are difficult to control. Instead: use paste. Or heat oven to 200 degrees, turn off, leave small dish of ammonia in oven overnight, then wipe oven with damp cloth and baking soda. Do not put baking soda on heating elements.
Toilet bowl cleaner	Corrosive. May be fatal if swallowed. *Toxicity 3–4˙*	Use up according to label instructions or wash down the sink or toilet with lots of water.	Ventilate room. Instead: use ordinary cleanser or detergent and baking soda.

Chemical Hazards in the Garage and Workshop

Product	Possible Hazards	Disposal Suggestions	Precautions and Substitutes
Aerosols	When sprayed, contents are broken into particles small enough to be inhaled. Cans may explode or burn.	Put **only** empty cans in trash. Do not burn. Do not place in trash compactor.	Store in cool place. Propellant may be flammable. Instead: use non-aerosol products.
Auto: antifreeze	Very poisonous. Has sweet taste—attractive to small children & pets. *Toxicity 3–4˙*	Amounts of less than 1 gallon pour down sink with plenty of water. Do **not** do this if you have a septic tank. Put in a secure container & take to a garage or service station.	No substitutes. Clean up any leaks or spills carefully.
Auto: batteries	Contain strong acid. Very corrosive. Danger to eyes & skin.	Recycle.	No substitutes. Trade in old batteries.
Auto: degreasers	Corrosive. Poisonous. Eye & skin irritant. *Toxicity 2–4˙*	Use up according to label instructions.	Choose strong detergent type over solvent type.
Auto: motor oil & transmission fluid	Poisonous. May be contaminated with lead. Skin & eye irritant.	Recycle.	No substitutes.
Paint strippers, thinners, & other solvents	Many are flammable. Eye & skin irritant. Moderately to very poisonous. *Toxicity 3–4˙*	Let settle, pour off cleaner for re-use. Pour sludge into container & seal, or wrap well in newspaper & throw in trash. Use up according to label instructions or save for hazardous waste collection day.	Avoid aerosols. Buy only as much as you need. Ventilate area well. Do not use near open flame. Instead of paint stripper: sand or use heat gun. Use water cleanup products as much as possible.
Paints, oil-based, & varnishes	Flammable. Eye & skin irritant. Use in small, closed area may cause unconsciousness.	Use up according to label instructions or save for hazardous waste collection day.	Ventilate area well. Do not use near open flame. May take weeks for fumes to go away. Instead: use water-based paints if possible.
Pesticides˙˙, herbicides, fungicides, slugbait, rodent poison, wood preservatives	All are dangerous to some degree. Can cause central nervous system damage, kidney & liver damage, birth defects, internal bleeding, eye injury. Some are readily absorbed through the skin. *Toxicity 3–6˙*	Use up carefully, following label instructions. Save for hazardous waste collection day.	Do not buy more than you need. Instead: try hand-picking, mechanical cultivation, natural predators. Practice good sanitation. Choose hardy varieties. Use insect lures & traps. As a last resort, use least toxic suitable pesticides.

*General Toxicity Rating

Number Rating	1	2	3	4	5	6
Toxicity Rating	Almost Non-Toxic	Slightly Toxic	Moderately Toxic	Very Toxic	Extremely Toxic	Super Toxic
Lethal Dose for 150 lb. Adult	More than 1 Quart	1 Pint to 1 Quart	1 Ounce to 1 Pint	1 Teaspoon to 1 Ounce	7 Drops to 1 Teaspoon	Less Than 7 Drops

For more information, contact your local public works department, hazardous waste agency, or poison control center.

**The following pesticides previously sold for use by homeowners and the general public have since been banned, or are no longer recommended for use by homeowners:

- Aldrin
- Arsenate
- Calcium Arsenate
- Chlordane
- Copper Arsenate

- Creosote
- DDT
- Dieldrin
- Heptachlor

- Pentachlorophenol (PCP)
- Silvex
- Sodium Arsenite
- 2-4-5T

If you have any of these pesticides, carefully store and save them for a hazardous waste collection day. Get a plastic container with a lid. (A five-gallon plastic bucket is ideal.) Fill the bucket halfway with cat litter. Keep the pesticide in its original container and put it in the bucket. Fill the bucket to the top with cat litter. Put the lid on it. Mark the container clearly, and store it on a shelf away from children and pets.

Source: Reprinted from the Illinois Hazardous Waste Research and Information Center.

tential for devastation, because in addition to poisoning individual users, they can pollute the environment if improperly disposed of—in effect, poisoning the entire planet. Toxic products include herbicides and insecticides.

Many household products have multiple potential for damage; that is, they fit into more than one of the foregoing categories. Aerosols, for instance, can explode if improperly disposed of. They also disperse sometimes dangerous substances into particles small enough to be inhaled. And some chemicals in aerosol propellants destroy the earth's ozone layer.

Obviously, we need many hazardous substances in our everyday lives. But safe substitutes are available for many harmful household chemicals. Baking soda, for example, can be substituted for many harmful kitchen and bathroom cleansers.

Unfortunately, no safe substitutes exist for certain hazardous substances. In these cases, safe use and disposal practices, including recycling, can minimize the dangers such chemicals pose to you and the environment.

The National Safety Council urges you to consider the health and safety of yourself, your community, and the environment every time you use a hazardous household substance. Be a smart consumer. Read product labels to find out how dangerous a substance is. If you can find a nonhazardous substitute for a hazardous product, do so. Otherwise, buy only the amount you need and then use it up or give the excess to someone who can use it.

Recycle as many harmful substances as possible. If you can't recycle, be sure to follow proper disposal procedures. Improper disposal of hazardous chemicals can injure trash collectors, other waste management personnel, and the environment. After solid garbage is collected, it is sent to municipal landfills. Eventually, chemicals in landfills can erode protective liners and enter the local groundwater. Certain liquid chemicals cannot be adequately treated by wastewater facilities. Liquid chemicals that end up in septic tanks often seep through and contaminate local groundwater. Throwing some hazardous substances into the trash or down the drain can have a devastating effect on lakes, rivers, and drinking water supplies. If you need to dispose of a hazardous chemical in your home, and the product label does not give disposal advice, call your local public health or sanitation department. They will explain how to dispose of the substance, or tell you when your community's next hazardous waste collection day will be.

Modern technology has brought us many advances but, in the process, it also has brought us to a threshold of danger. The chemical substances we have come to rely on for our existence may be the agents of our destruction. Proper use of these substances is our responsibility. Our future, as individuals and as a global community, depends on it.

Source: *Healthline,* February 1990, pp. 11–13.

Read the labels of all substances brought into the home. If they are toxic, lock them up so that children cannot get to them. Although medications are often kept in child-resistant containers, they should also be locked away; children often show great ingenuity in opening those childproof caps.

Grandparents need to maintain these precautions as well. A recent study by the American Association of Poison Control Centers found that grandparents do not always keep their medications in child-resistant containers or locked up. One out of 6 poisoning cases involving medications, in fact, occurs in the grandparents' home when the grandchild is visiting.

If an accidental poisoning occurs in the home, taking the proper action can be critical to the survival of the victim. The procedures listed below should be followed:

1. Call the nearest Poison Control Center, physician, or hospital for instructions. These numbers can be found by checking the blue pages of the telephone book, calling directory assistance, or dialing 911. Keep all emergency numbers posted near the telephone. Emergency numbers can also be programmed into telephones that have a memory feature.

   Syrup of ipecac: A liquid medication derived from the ipecac plant; used to induce vomiting when a poisoning has occurred; also known as ipecacuanha.

2. Keep **syrup of ipecac, activated charcoal,** and **epsom salts** on hand, but use them only on the advice of a physician or poison control center.

   Activated charcoal: A highly absorbent form of carbon that is used as an antidote for certain types of poisons.

For more information on preventing poisoning, contact:

Institute of Education Communications
Children's Hospital of Pittsburgh
3705 Fifth Avenue at DeSoto Street
Pittsburgh, PA 15213

Epsom salts: A bitter, colorless salt consisting of hydrated magnesium sulfate that is used to induce vomiting when poisoning has occurred.

FIREARMS

Statistics show that a household gun is 12 times more likely to kill a friend or relative than an intruder.

Almost 60 percent of the approximately 2,400 accidental deaths caused by firearms in this country each year occur in and around the home. More than one-fourth of these victims are under the age of 14.

Improper storage, careless handling, and poor cleaning practices are factors in most of the deaths. Many firearms accidents occur when people handle guns without knowing they are loaded. Many injuries and deaths have occurred when children, handling real guns as though they were toys, have playfully pulled the trigger.

Anyone possessing firearms should observe the following rules:

1. Keep guns and all firearms locked up and out of the reach of children.

2. Do not keep a loaded gun in the house.

3. Store guns and ammunition separately.

4. Do not handle a gun, or allow a gun in the house, before checking to see if it is loaded. Check both the chamber and the magazine.

5. Never point a gun—loaded or unloaded—at anyone.

6. Take a firearms safety course that teaches how to clean and handle a gun.

ELECTRICAL SHOCK

Electricity helps make the modern American home efficient and comfortable. It provides lighting and powers a multitude of household appliances and tools. Most of the time it poses no hazard to its users. In certain circumstances, however, household electricity can pose a serious danger.

It is important to be aware of the risks associated with electricity. After receiving a slight shock from a malfunctioning hair dryer or toaster, many people conclude that household current is basically harmless. That is not the case, however. Under the right circumstances, even the small amount of current required to run an electric toothbrush (10 watts) can kill a person.

The "right circumstances" often involve moisture. An **electric current** is always traveling toward the ground and will follow the path of least resistance toward that destination. Dry human skin offers a large amount of resistance to current and will allow only a small amount of electricity to flow through the body. A small amount of moisture, however, can change that situation dramatically. Sweaty skin, for example, is much less resistant to electricity and will conduct enough current to cause serious injury or death. A person in contact with a puddle on the floor or with water in a bathtub or sink **conducts** current like a lightning rod. Any appliance that falls into a bathtub will instantly **electrocute** the bather.

Electrical cords and wiring present a special hazard to young children who may be tempted to chew them. Even the small amount of moisture present in a child's mouth is enough to cause household current to flow through the body, leading to serious injury or death.

Following these basic rules will greatly reduce the risk of suffering electrical injury:

1. Use 3-prong grounded plugs. The third prong cuts off the current if there is an electrical leak. Some new power tools are double-insulated and do not require 3-prong grounded plugs. They are very safe unless immersed in water or exposed to rain.

2. Place safety plugs in all sockets to protect children from the hazards of an unused electrical outlet.

3. Keep all extension cords well hidden—out of the reach of children.

4. Do not use electric appliances or tools around water or while standing in water.

5. Use only electrical appliances and tools that bear the approval stamp of the Underwriters Laboratories (UL).

6. Do not overload circuits.

For additional suggestions, see the box entitled "Nine Electrical Hazards at Home."

Emergency Treatment for Electrical Shock

The severity of an electrical shock is largely determined by the length of time the current flows through the body. The longer the

(continued on p. 64)

Electric current: A flow of charged electrons.

Conduct: To transmit electricity; materials that have the ability to conduct electricity are known as conductors.

Electrocute: To kill by electric shock.

Nine Electrical Hazards at Home

When you think of electrical hazards, shock and electrocution might come to mind. Although these are important dangers to guard against, two other potential electrical hazards exist around your home: fire and burns. When checking your home against electrical hazards, consider all of these potential dangers. To help you locate problems in your home, here are [9] common household electrical hazards and their potential dangers.

1. OVERLOADED WALL OUTLETS

Do your wall and extension-cord outlets have so many adapters, plugs, and cords protruding that they resemble octopuses? These so-called "octopus connections" are dangerous. You may hear warnings about the multiple use of an outlet, but do you know why?

If you plug too many electrical products into one outlet, you're trying to pull more electricity through the wires that lead to the outlet than the wires are equipped to handle. It's as if you were trying to rush a crowd of people through a hallway and out the doorway on the other end. If only one or two people exit at a time, there's no problem. But if everyone pushes through at once, the hall and doorway become overcrowded as people jostle each other.

With an overloaded electrical wire, too many electrons move through the wire at once. As they jostle each other and push through the wire, resistance builds. As a result, the wire heats up. This creates danger because the hot wire can start a fire. Fires from over-loaded circuits usually start within your home's walls and can produce a high amount of heat before flames actually break out. By the time you know there's a fire, you may not have time to do anything about it.

If you find yourself with more plugs than outlets, ask an electrician to evaluate your home's wiring system. The electrician may suggest adding outlets or upgrading the wiring or both. Just as more doorways and larger hallways lessen the resistance in the people-rush example, more wall outlets and higher-capacity wires can reduce resistance in your home's electrical system.

2. MISUSED PLUGS AND ADAPTERS

Misuse of polarized plugs, three-pronged plugs, or three-pronged outlet adapters can lead to electrical shock.

Newer plugs (and plug outlets) have one side wider than the other. (This is called polarization.) Polarized plugs help prevent electrical shock. The wider blade of the plug is designed to fit into only the wider slot of the wall or extension-cord outlet, which is considered the "neutral" side. Electricity flows from the narrow side, which is attached to the "hot" or "live" wire. The "hot" wire will be attached to the switch, so it may be switched off. Similarly, the inside shell of a lamp outlet will be attached to the "neutral" wire to prevent shock during bulb replacement.

If you have to push especially hard to fit a plug into an outlet, check to see whether the plug is polarized. If it is, be sure the outlet is also polarized. And be sure you insert the plug correctly so that the wide blade fits into the wide slot. Never force a polarized plug into a non-polarized outlet, and don't attempt to trim the wide blade to fit into a narrow slot. If your wall outlets are not polarized, an expert needs to replace them, or you can investigate the use of an appropriate adapter. If your extension cord is not polarized, buy a new one and make sure it has a polarized cord.

The purpose of three-pronged plugs is to send any possible short circuit down the third wire to the ground. If you don't have the third prong plugged into a grounded outlet, you could receive a dangerous shock. If you must use an extension cord with an electrical product that has a three-pronged plug, be sure to use a three-wire cord of proper capacity for the product. (Ask your hardware dealer to match the gauge, amperage, voltage, and watt capacity of the cord to the requirements of your electrical product.)

If you use a three-prong adapter, buy one with a metal tab that fits under the screw of the wall outlet cover plate. (Old adapters with "pigtail" wires are more dangerous to use.) Always be sure the tab is connected to the wall-plate screw. If you think your wiring is not properly grounded, ask an electrician to check out your entire electrical system.

3. WORN, CRACKED CORDS AND PLUGS
Check all cords, plugs and extension-cord outlets periodically to be sure they're not worn or cracked. A worn or cracked cord, plug, or outlet can cause electrical shock if touched and can short-circuit, producing heat and eventual fire. Hire an expert to replace worn or cracked cords and plugs on electrical appliances, and discard worn or cracked extension cords. Never attempt a "stop-gap" repair by using electrical tape.

4. TWISTED, KNOTTED, DANGEROUSLY PLACED CORDS
Twisted or knotted cords can quickly lead to worn, cracked cords. And the worn or cracked portion can hide within the twist or knot of the cord. Iron cords often have this problem. Check all cords that are twisted, and straighten and untangle any twisted or knotted cords. (Remember to check cords behind your furniture, as well.)

Dangerously placed cords can result in wear or can cause an accident. To prevent wear and possible tripping accidents, don't run cords along the floor in doorways or other traffic areas. Similarly, don't hang cords—even temporarily—where a passing adult, child or pet could become caught up in them. There's the added danger that a person might pull an electrical product down and on top of himself or herself. Consider the burns or bruises possible from a surprise tug on an electrical cord attached to an electric frying pan, iron, power tool, or other heavy electrical product!

Electrical cords should not be wrapped around or draped over steam pipes, furnaces, heaters or any other hot surface. The heat can scorch or dry out the cord's insulation, and possible shock or short-circuit fire can result.

5. OPEN OUTLETS
If you have young children or visiting youngsters in your home, use "safety caps" on all unused plug outlets—in both wall outlets and extension cords. Toddlers are especially likely to touch an open hole with a finger or paper clip, for example, and cause serious electrical shock.

Also, unplug and remove unused extension cords. Crawling babies and infants in the chewing stage are often attracted to extension cords and may "mouth" or chew on the outlet end. If the cord is plugged in, the mouth's saliva can set up a short circuit between the metal portions of the cord outlet. The short circuit can quickly produce high heat and result in potentially severe burns to the soft parts of a child's mouth. Such burns can cause lifelong scars.

6. PLUGGED-IN APPLIANCES
Most instruction booklets included with small kitchen appliances warn not to leave appliances plugged in while not in use. If an unused appliance is left plugged in, there is still electricity attached to it. And shocks can occur when you touch the appliance.

Thermostat controls on appliances such as irons, electric frying pans, and electric ovens don't always provide a complete off setting. Also, plugged-in appliances can be accidentally turned on. Cuts, burns, overheating, and fire can occur. A removable thermostat cord left plugged in and resting on a countertop can cause shocks if you touch it; it can also short-circuit if you spill water or allow water to leak around and under it.

When you finish using an electric appliance or power tool, follow these three steps (in this order): (1) turn the appliance off; (2) unplug the appliance from the wall outlet (hold the plug but don't tug at it); (3) if the appliance has a removable cord, remove the cord from the appliance.

7. BATHROOM APPLIANCES
Although bathroom appliances (hair driers, electric toothbrushes, and shaver, for instance) are usually manufactured to protect against electric shock, you still need to handle them carefully. Keep other appliances, such as electric radios and clocks, away from water and far from the reach of wet hands.

A plugged-in bathroom appliance can cause shock and even electrocution if it falls into a water-filled sink, the shower, or a filled bathtub. Keep such appliances away from the sink, shower, and tub. Remember to unplug them when you're done or if you leave the objects unattended.

An electric hair drier can also cause burns—even at medium heat—when used by children or on babies and infants, who sometimes can't tell you how hot the heat is. The solution is not to use hair driers on babies and infants. Use only with caution on young children and on pets.

Be sure your hands and feet are dry before you reach to turn off, turn on, pick up, or otherwise adjust any plugged-in appliance. Place appliances, such as radios or televisions, so they're inconvenient to touch while someone is using water.

8. FLAMMABLE MATERIALS
Keep flammable gases, liquids, clothing, curtains, and paper away from electric plugs, switches, and heating and cooking appliances. A spark from unplugging a plug or turning a switch on or off can be enough to ignite flammable gases and some flammable liquids. Take care in workshop areas to keep electrical appliances away from flammable gases and liquids.

Also, keep electrical products away from flammable materials elsewhere in the house. For example, grease and oil (as well as grease- and oil-soaked trash) should neither be kept nor stored near an electric frying pan. Likewise, don't hang flammable curtains above the stove or a paper-towel holder above the electric oven or toaster. Avoid wearing loose-fitting and flammable clothing while you cook.

Even light bulbs produce enough heat to start fires. Don't drape paper or cloth over a lamp or bare bulb. Most electric appliances generate heat; therefore, keep them away from flammable materials and place them where they get adequate ventilation to prevent overheating.

9. WASHERS AND DRIERS
It's especially important to properly ground electric washers and driers according to manufacturers' specifications. Your chances of having wet hands and feet (or even standing in water) are more likely in a laundry room. Therefore, be sure you properly ground laundry appliances to prevent a serious shock.

You may want to consider replacing your washer and drier electric outlets with GFCIs (ground fault circuit interrupters). A GFCI is designed to cut the power if it detects an electrical leak from the circuit, thus keeping you from becoming the "ground" through which the electricity passes. You can use GFCIs to replace outlets where shock is likely to occur (laundry room, kitchen, bathroom, damp basements, garages, and outdoor outlets). Or you can wire GFCIs into circuits at the panel box. Be sure to follow the manufacturer's directions, which include the periodic testing of the GFCI.

Source: National Safety Council, reprinted in *Healthline*, April 1991, pp. 4–6.

exposure, the more serious the injury and the greater the likelihood of death.

If you witness an electric shock you should act immediately to cut off the electrical power or, if that is not possible, to separate the victim from the electrical source. Even a very small amount of current can cause the victim to freeze so that he or she cannot let go. If this happens, do not attempt to pull the person free with your bare hands; the current will enter your body as well. Instead use a piece of a nonconducting material such as wood to knock the person free.

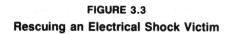

FIGURE 3.3
Rescuing an Electrical Shock Victim

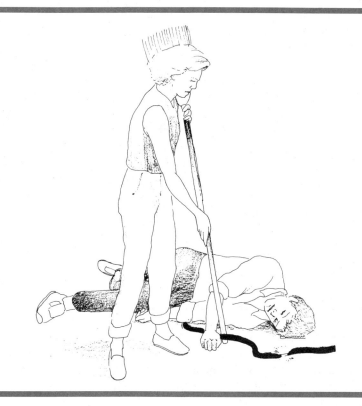

Do not touch a victim of electric shock until he or she is separated from the electrical source. If you are unable to turn off the power, pull or push the person away from the electrical source using a piece of material that does not conduct electricity, such as wood, rope, or fabric.

Electric shocks cause 2 types of injury: burns (both external and internal) and respiratory or **cardiac arrest**. When both are involved, the first priority should be to attempt to restore heartbeat and breathing. Applying **CPR** immediately can save the person's life. In the time that it takes for an ambulance to arrive, the victim could die.

Every victim of an electric shock should go to the hospital, even if there is no apparent injury. Electric burns are often more serious than they first appear.

Cardiac arrest: A halt in the pumping action of the heart caused by cessation of its rhythmic muscular activity.

CPR: Cardiopulmonary resuscitation; an emergency procedure used to treat someone who is not breathing or whose heart has stopped beating by applying a combination of external cardiac massage and rescue breathing.

OTHER HOME HAZARDS

Gunshot wounds, electric shocks, inadvertent poisonings, and falls are the most prevalent types of home accidents, but other potential hazards merit precautions.

Ladders

Every year falls from ladders cause numerous injuries that could be prevented. When extra height is needed to bring an object within reach, always use a ladder rather than a box or some other unsteady object, but make sure to select the right ladder.

As a general rule, an extension ladder should be 4 feet longer than the height that needs to be reached. The last 3 rungs are not meant to be used and may not provide adequate support. Most ladders list a maximum weight they can support. This weight should not be exceeded.

When an extension ladder is used to reach a roof, the ladder should extend at least 3 feet above the roof or gutter. This provides a railing to grasp when climbing on or off the roof. Do not use a ladder that is not in excellent condition. Make sure it is properly secured at the base before climbing it. If the ground is soft, place a plank under the ladder's feet to prevent it from sinking.

Metal is an excellent conductor of electrical current, and high tension wires carry many times the amount of current needed to kill a human. When a metal ladder meets a wire, the shock can be deadly. It is best to use wooden or fiberglass ladders around high tension wires.

Lawn Mowers

Another widely used piece of equipment around the yard is the power lawn mower. Unfortunately it can also be one of the most hazardous. The Consumer Product Safety Commission estimates that more than 50,000 people are treated every year for injuries caused by power mowers. About 68 percent of those injuries are caused when the operator's hand or foot comes in contact with the rotating blade, and another 20 percent are caused when objects are thrown from the blades and hit either the operator or someone nearby.

Mowing a wet lawn, especially on rough or steep terrain, can be particularly dangerous. The chance of slipping and coming in contact with the blades greatly increases on wet grass. Soggy turf also clogs the blades or discharge chutes and may have to be

FIGURE 3.4
Mowing Safety

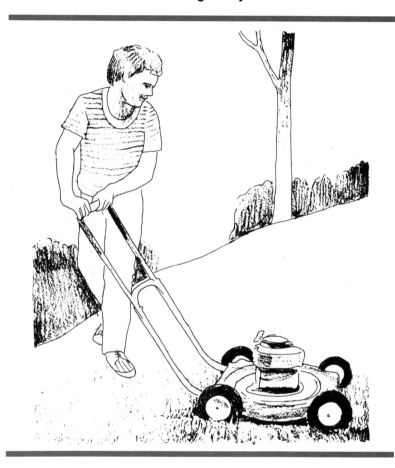

Mowing the lawn on steep terrain can be hazardous. When using a hand mower, mow horizontally across the slope. It is also advisable to wear ear protectors and shoes with soles that will not slip.

Did You Know That . . .

Old-style push (manual) lawn mowers have become more popular recently: they're less expensive than power models, less polluting—and less dangerous.

removed physically. This can be dangerous because manually turning the blades during the cleaning process may be enough to start the motor even if it has been turned off. It is important, therefore, not only to turn off the mower but to disconnect the spark plug before reaching into the blade housing to clean this area. In addition, never try to use an electric mower on a wet lawn; it can lead to a deadly electrical short.

Did You Know That . . .

Drowning is now the second leading cause of accidental death among children. Half of these deaths occur in home swimming pools.

Steep terrain also has special hazards. Using a riding mower on sloped embankments or steep areas, for instance, can lead to a rollover. The best way to avoid this mishap is to mow up and down the slope. A hand mower, however, should never be pushed up and down, because it can slip backwards and hit the mower's feet. A safer approach is to mow horizontally across the slope.

Wearing the proper clothing is the best protection from objects thrown by the blades. Sturdy shoes are especially important. Wear goggles when using weed whips or power hedgers.

Power Tools

The number of home workshops has increased in recent years and with them the number of accidents involving power tools. The most commonly used power tool is the electric drill, which accounts for approximately one-third of the injuries. Other tools that can cause injury are routers, grinders, lathes, saws, planers, glue guns, and grinders.

Most accidents occur when the handler inadvertently comes in contact with the blade, bit, or other revolving part of the tool. To ensure safety, make sure you are using the proper tool for the job, never put extra pressure on the tool, and make sure to read thoroughly and follow exactly the tool's operating instructions.

Swimming Pools

Drownings often occur in backyard pools when young children wander alone into an unattended pool or when they are momentarily left at the pool unsupervised. In order to prevent these tragedies, make sure all children are under *constant* supervision when in the pool area. A child who falls into an unattended pool can drown in a matter of 2–3 minutes and seldom, if ever, is able to cry out. In addition, enclose the pool area in a 6-foot fence with a self-closing, self-locking gate to keep children out during other times.

Suffocation

In the United States, approximately 3,000 deaths each year, many in the home, are caused by **suffocation**. [4] Almost half of the victims are children under the age of 5. Young children are susceptible to suffocation for a number of reasons.

First, babies explore their environments by putting things in their mouths, including small items that they can accidentally swallow and that can cut off their oxygen. The best way to prevent this kind of mishap is to keep small objects, including pins, buttons, coins, screws, and toys, off the floor and out of the reach of infants and toddlers.

Suffocation: A lack of oxygen caused by obstruction of the passageways that carry air into the lungs.

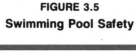

FIGURE 3.5
Swimming Pool Safety

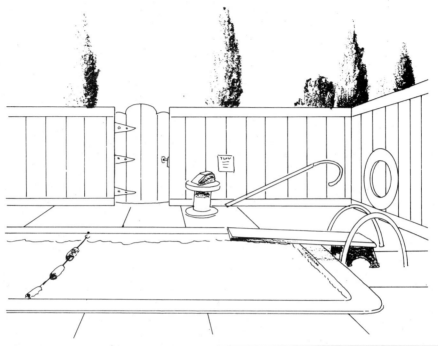

A pool area needs to be enclosed with a fence with a self-closing, self-locking gate. Rescue equipment and a telephone should be located nearby.

Cribs are another danger area. Children can suffocate on bedding (especially plastic mattress covers), on pillows, and even on overly soft mattresses. Ill-fitting mattresses can leave a gap at the edge where a baby's head can become trapped, and toys strung above the crib at head height can cause strangulation. Parents must make sure their children's sleeping areas are safe from these dangers. Many experts recommend that parents keep their child's room warm enough so that blankets are not even necessary. Plastic bedding and pillows of any kind should also be avoided.

Large airtight appliances such as refrigerators, freezers, and picnic coolers have also contributed to the suffocation death toll.

(continued on p. 74)

Safe at Home

I used to think of my home as a sort of refuge, a safe harbor in a perilous world. Life's significant hazards were either invisible, like radon, or somewhere else. When I was away I worried about drunk drivers, frayed elevator cables, and exploding airplanes. At home I could relax. Now, thanks to a booklet put out by the National Safety Council, I'm somewhat less sanguine about this creaky old two-story Victorian. The booklet is called *Accident Facts*. I picked it up at the doctor's office while waiting to have some stitches removed from my thumb, which I'd sliced deeply with a paring knife.

According to the Safety Council, some 20 million people were injured at home in 1987—about one in eleven Americans. Every three seconds, on a typical day, someone else falls victim. By midnight tonight, 56 of them will be dead or dying.

Right now I'm at home myself, pecking at the personal computer in my study. Two extension cords cohabit the single electrical outlet. One runs to the computer, even though the instruction manual explicitly recommends a direct connection to the outlet. The other extension cord has just two prongs and a coppery glint where the plug is pulling loose. This cord sends current to the desk lamp, the electric pencil sharpener, the phone answering machine, and the clock. Oh, and the space heater, too, which is at the moment casting a rosy glow on a pile of old newspapers, manuscripts, and other highly flammable printed matter.

You could say I work in a firetrap. The National Safety Council might say my study should be condemned. Yet I wouldn't have to do much to make it a safe place to be. In a world beset by dangers, every home is still a haven in one respect: Most home accidents can be prevented—with a *little* common sense, that is.

You just need to recall a few crucial tricks and make some simple but significant improvements. Which steps you choose to take, of course, depends on whom you live with. Households with

toddlers require features that become obsolete once the kids grow up a bit. Older folks face a completely different set of perils.

The Accidental Resident: A Review

Fire!

If you're like me, you always figured the only house fire you'd ever see was on the TV news. Dreadful things like that just don't happen to rational, responsible people, right?

I've got news for you: [In 1988] there were 538,500 home fires, claiming almost 5,000 victims. Seventeen-year-old Sean Studer, who lives not far from me, was very nearly one of them.

On a Wednesday in mid-August Sean woke to the sound of shattering glass. It didn't take him long to get the picture: Hot, gray smoke was pouring under the door, while down in the driveway his buddy Jay Schoeller was yelling and heaving big rocks at his window. (He'd been outside working on a car the two were rebuilding.) Sean held his breath, flung open the door, and bolted downstairs into the smoke. He crawled out the front door and was quickly joined on the lawn by his twin sisters, aged 16. Shannon had also escaped through the front door, but Erin had climbed out a window, lowered herself till she was hanging by her fingertips, then dropped to the walkway ten feet below.

Sean's mind raced. His father was at work—but his mother? The house was already a torch! Jay pointed out that her car was not in the garage.

Kathleen Studer, it turns out, had fixed herself some toast for breakfast, then gone out to run errands. The Studers later told fire chief Dan Winkel that the toaster had been acting up the day before, sparking and making popping sounds. They now speculate that a broken heating wire inside the toaster ignited a slice of toast left in one slot. The flames apparently then spread to some paper napkins and a cloth toaster cover lying on the counter nearby. Winkel's fire crew arrived within 15 minutes of

Sean's escape, but not before most of the house had burned. In the words of one firefighter, the Studer children came within "an angel's breath" of not getting out in time.

From the moment open flames appear, it takes only one minute for smoke, toxic gases, and heat to rise to the ceiling and begin radiating downward. After two minutes the room heats to the kindling temperature of the furniture, and everything goes up. After just two more minutes, the whole house is ablaze. Early warning, obviously, can mean the difference between life and death.

You know about smoke detectors, of course. You've probably had them for years. But when was the last time you checked them? The National Fire Protection Association says the odds are that 1) they're in the wrong place; 2) you need more; or 3) they need new batteries. (Eighty-two percent of all American homes have smoke detectors, but at least a third of those aren't working properly.)

Test your smoke detectors often. (Expect to change the batteries at least once a year.) Detectors should be placed in every major living area—at least one per floor in central locations—away from air vents, either on the ceiling or below the ceiling on the wall, at least four to 12 inches from any right angle. If you ever have reason to remodel, replace all battery-powered smoke detectors with ones wired into your home's circuitry. They're more reliable. (In some states these are now mandatory in new homes.)

Plan escape routes. Draw a floor plan of your home and map two ways out of every room. Have family members memorize the plan, then, when everyone's in bed, push the "test" button on one of the alarms. If the house isn't empty in less than a minute, repeat the drill until it is. Choose a meeting place outside so you can count heads.

If a fire starts, get everyone out first. Then—no matter how small the blaze—reach for a telephone, not a fire extinguisher, the garden hose, or a bucket. Your neighbor's phone is a far better choice than your own, but hedge your bets: Is the fire department's number right beside each of your phones? If not, put it there now. And while you're at it, write down the number of the poison control center, the police department, your family doctor, and a relative or neighbor who can be called in an emergency.

Clean beneath your stove burners. Of course it sounds silly, but when fire breaks out in the kitchen, the main culprit is most often plain old grease that someone ignored.

The Appliances' Revenge
Electrical wiring and appliances will cause tens of thousands of home fires this year. A sixth of all home-fire deaths are caused by heating equipment, often electric space heaters. Extension cords are especially troublesome, probably because they're so often abused and overloaded.

More than a year ago Underwriters Laboratory removed its seal of approval from all light-duty extension cords except those equipped with a circuit breaker or fuse in the plug. Many of the lightweight two-prong extension cords you see in supermarkets and hardware stores would fail this stringent new standard. Don't be misled by the UL label—these were made before the change. When the old ones run out this model will be extinct.

Unplug all the extension cords in your home and pile them on the living room floor. Get a pair of wirecutters, bite your lip, then cut in two and throw away any light, two-prong cord without a built-in circuit breaker. Replace it with the new kind.

Turn on everything plugged into each extension cord, wait an hour, then feel the cord. If it's hot, it could start a fire. Here's how: Heated cord insulation can harden and crumble, or it can melt, allowing the wires to meet, spark, and ignite things nearby. The insulating plastic on an overloaded extension cord melts at about 250°.

Reroute any extension cord that's stapled to the wall or running under a carpet or through a doorway—the prime locations for cord abuse. A cord that's cracked, crushed, spliced, or otherwise disfigured is a hazard. (Don't try to mend it—buy a new one. Or better yet, rearrange things so you don't need *any* extension cords.)

Remember the three-foot rule the next time you plug in a space heater. The heater's front grill must be at least three feet away from *anything,* flammable or not.

On The Cutting Edge

Ever slice yourself with a kitchen knife? According to the National Council, kitchen cutlery tops the list of hazardous household tools, causing more than 350,000 serious accidents in the home in 1987, more than twice the number blamed on glassware and eight times as many as caused by cooking ranges and ovens combined. What's the most dangerous knife? Any one that's dull. A knife so blunt that it skids off an onion is still sharp enough to cut *you* on its path toward the cutting board.

Regularly test your knives for sharpness: Try slicing a wet tomato or green pepper, exerting only slight pressure. If the blade slides off or fails to bite instantly into the skin, the knife is dangerously dull.

Make sure your knives *stay* sharp. Empty your knife drawer and fill it with something else— napkins or hot pads. Give away any knife you don't use at least twice a week, and take the rest to a professional sharpener. Pick a new place to store them where the blades can never touch anything harder than wood or plastic and where you can see them when you reach for them. A wooden block on a shelf is ideal.

Got a Permit To Use That Ladder, Buddy?

You probably know someone like my friend Phil Brown.* He's a handy guy, good with tools. But impulsive. Last month he felt the urge to hang a South American textile over the mantel in his living room, which happens to have a two-story, vaulted ceiling. He got out the extension ladder and prudently asked his wife to hold the base while he climbed up—ignoring the fact that he'd planted the ladder's feet on a loose carpet. "Could you hand me that hammer?" he asked. She let go, and instantly the ladder's base skidded away from the wall, kicking pleats into the carpet as it picked up speed. Miraculously, he only bruised his left hip and a finger.

Ladders will be implicated in more than 100,000 home accidents this year. But you're not

* A pseudonym.

like Phil Brown. You know how to use a ladder. Which means, of course, that you always follow the four-to-one rule? And the three-foot overlap rule? Sure you do.

For every four feet up, plant a ladder's feet one foot out from the supporting wall. That places the ladder at the most stable angle.

Always allow three feet of overlap at the top. Suppose you're checking your roof, the edge of which is ten feet up. The ladder must be more than 13 feet long, so that at least three feet of ladder can extend above the point of contact with the roofline. That way you'll have a secure handle when stepping from the ladder to the roof and back again.

When using a folding stepladder, never, ever stand on the top two rungs. Turn an empty glass upside down on your kitchen table. Balance on it a full bottle of soda or beer—upside down, on its cap. Unstable? That's you standing on the topmost rung of a stepladder.

Toddlers Without Trauma

I know, I know. *Your* kids are absolutely secure at home; you never let them out of your sight. Well, listen to this: While I looked on—paralyzed with disbelief—my 9-month-old daughter rammed her walker through a sturdy-looking gate at the head of our stairs and tumbled the whole way down. She only lost two teeth, but she could have died. Falls are a major cause of accidental death in kids aged one to four. When it comes to catastrophic mishaps, poisonings join them near the top of the list.

Running Fence

Stair gates are not an option for families with small children: They're a must. They belong at the top *and* bottom of staircases. When there's a gate only at the top, a child may climb halfway up, then panic when he or she realizes the difficulty of the descent. Gates also belong on doors leading outside or to the garage.

Spring-loaded or pressure-mounted gates that aren't permanently fastened at one end are unreliable, and crisscross accordion-style gates can collapse under pressure and trap a toddler's head. Best are sliding gates, which open and close like a patio door.

Test the security of each gate. Does it have a working latch? Could a child push it open? Would it stop a toddler on a rolling red wagon or skateboard? If not, buy a better one. (About walkers: They may help babies learn to walk, but they give them a mobility that far exceeds their judgment. Let 'em crawl.)

Bet that any child tall enough to reach a doorknob knows how to open it. Fit a plastic sleeve (from the hardware store) over the knob on the door to the basement stairs. Only your firm adult grip can turn it now.

Close gaps in railing and banisters. Buy some $^1/_{16}$-inch-thick clear plastic panels at your local home center, and while you're there pick up some nylon "cable ties" to fasten the panels to the banisters through holes in the panels at both top and bottom.

Check for other hazards, especially the windows. (A child can fall through a five-inch opening, and don't count on the window screen to stop him.) Fasten safety locks on the upper tracks of double-hung windows so they can open no more than four inches. Install door-type safety chains on side-hinged casement windows and clamp-on stops on sliding windows.

Pretty Poisons

The good news is, relatively few children actually *die* from overdoses of antibiotics, aspirin, bathroom cleaner, charcoal lighter, dishwashing detergent, gasoline, glue, insecticides, lye, nail polish, oven cleaner, paint thinner, pesticides, rat poison, rubbing alcohol, shoe polish, vitamins, or any other of the hundreds of toxic substances common in the average home. The bad news: This year there'll be 1.2 million accidental poisonings, two-thirds of which will involve children.

You're certainly well aware of the hazards of cleaning agents like Tilex (active ingredient: sodium hypochlorite). But did you know that a little bottle of vanilla extract contains enough alcohol to knock a toddler out cold? Or that one bottle of minty mouthwash has the same alcoholic punch as a whole bottle of wine? Or that antifreeze and windshield cleaner—both deadly poisons—have an appealing sweet taste? Or that for a small child the toxic dose of Extra-strength Tylenol

(active ingredient: acetaminophen) is just five tablets?

If you suspect your child has been poisoned, immediately call the local poison control center. *Don't give the child anything without advice from the center or a doctor.* The most common treatment is to induce vomiting with a spoonful of syrup of ipecac (always have a bottle at home). But if your child has swallowed a corrosive cleaner, such as lye, which might burn the esophagus if vomited, activated charcoal may be prescribed. More effective than syrup of ipecac, charcoal "absorbs" the poison, binding it before it can get to the intestinal tract.

Securing your storage cupboards will greatly cut the risk of poisoning in your home.

Put plastic padlock-style safety devices on all storage cabinets with knobs or pulls, pressure-release latches on cabinets that don't have knobs, and spring loaded safety latches on drawers. (Ask for these at a hardware store.)

Move medicines from the bathroom medicine chest or vanity to a high, latched cabinet.

Check the caps on your medications. In a 1986 survey of nine poison control centers, 65 percent of the child-resistant packages they'd collected after poisonings were found to be working improperly. (Children's Liquid Tylenol and many other kids' medicines are made to taste good. Keep them well hidden and don't ever refer to them as candy.)

Retirement Without Risks

My grandmother lived her whole life in a big old house with two steep staircases and a huge clawfoot tub in the main bathroom. As she grew older, keeping her house became an obsession that prompted her to walk every day, eat well, and keep an active mind. But in her 90s her vision and hearing began to fail, and one morning she slipped and fell hard while getting out of the tub. She was only bruised, but that one accident shattered her confidence. She drained her savings to pay a full-time nurse and never lived independently again.

The elderly suffer more serious domestic mishaps than any other age group. They account for a third of all deaths in home fires. Falls are even more insidious killers. Seventy percent of fatal falls are taken by those 65 or over. Broken hips are common. Each year 200,000 people over age 45 suffer hip fractures. In one study of elderly men and women hospitalized with broken hips, only half were able to return home again to live. Don't wait for that discouraging first fall.

Secure the edges of throw rugs and loose carpets with double-face adhesive carpet tape. Reroute any extension cord that crosses a passageway. Inspect fully for exposed nails, frayed staircase runners, and loose metal threshold trim (where carpet or linoleum run up to the edge of hardwood flooring, for instance).

Install railings on both sides of all stairways, and grab bars in the bathroom beside the toilet and over the bathtub. Paint them in bold, contrasting colors.

Replace all low-wattage light bulbs with the brightest bulbs the lamp or fixture will take. Older people may require three times as much light as do younger people. If a lamp or fixture won't handle at least 100 watts, replace it with one that will.

Test all tables for their ability to support an adult. Stand beside the table, place your palms on its surface, and slowly shift your full weight from your feet to your hands. If the table tilts, sways, or creaks loudly, move it away from daily foot traffic. Better yet, give it away (card tables should be the first to go).

Source: Bonnie Blodgett, *Hippocrates* (November/December 1989), pp. 57–60.

Children sometimes crawl into them while playing and become trapped.

Home accidents take a high toll among the elderly and the young. Fortunately, a good home safety awareness program can prevent almost all potentially fatal mishaps. The time and knowledge it takes to make a home safe will pay high dividends for the entire family. W

Outdoor Accidents

4

OUTDOOR RECREATION has become almost an American obsession. Vacationers eager for fun and relaxation flock to beaches, campgrounds, and wooded areas whenever they have the chance. But this outdoor activity explosion has brought an increase in outdoor accidents. In the rush to have a good time, vacationers often forget safety.

WATER SPORTS

Water activities, which attract more than 100 million participants each year, are the most popular form of outdoor sports in America. They also can be deadly. Drownings claim 7,000 lives every year, and 70,000 are involved in near-drownings. For adults under the age of 45, only automobile accidents claim more lives. Unfortunately almost half of the participants lack the basic skill required to make water activities safe: They don't know how to swim.

Swimming
Every person who wants to participate in any type of water activity should learn to swim in a certified swimming program. Organizations that offer such programs in most communities include the American Red Cross, the local YMCA, and local schools.

Those who have not yet taken swimming lessons should learn a technique called **survival floating**. The technique is quite simple and easily learned. It involves learning to float in the water face down in a relaxed position with the arms hanging

(continued on p. 77)

Survival floating: A technique designed to help swimmers and non-swimmers alike survive in the water for extended periods of time. Developed during World War II for downed pilots, it minimizes the effort needed to breathe while floating in the water by taking advantage of the body's natural buoyancy.

FIGURE 4.1
Survival Floating

Step 1. The Resting Position

a) Take a deep breath and sink vertically.
b) Relax the body, letting your arms hang at your sides and your chin drop to your chest.

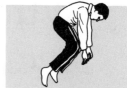

Step 2. Preparing to Breathe

a) Slowly lift your arms to shoulder height in front of your head.
b) Raise one knee toward the chest and extend the other leg behind your body in a striding position.

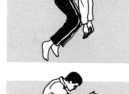

Step 3. Exhaling

a) Gently raise your head out of the water and exhale; your chin should still be in the water.

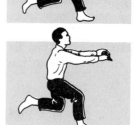

Step 4. Inhaling

a) Gently sweep your arms out and down while kicking gently downward with your feet; this will raise your body slightly higher in the water until the bottom of your chin is at or just above the surface.
b) Breathe in normally.

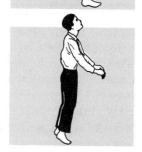

Step 5. Returning to the Resting Position

a) As you sink back down into the water, let your arms drop to your sides and relax your legs, allowing your feet to come together.
b) Drop your chin to your chest.

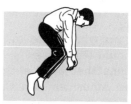

Survival floating, or "drown proofing," is a technique that utilizes the body's natural buoyancy to reduce to a minimum the effort required to survive in the water until rescued.

at your sides. From this position, the head can easily be lifted out of the water 5 or 6 times a minute to take deep breaths. Between breaths, the "swimmer" returns to the face-down float. Using this technique, depicted in figure 4.1, even a nonswimmer can survive in the water for an extended period of time with a minimum expenditure of energy.

Nonswimmers are not the only ones who can get in trouble in the water. Even strong swimmers can drown when they do not take proper precautions. Every swimmer, regardless of skill level, should observe the following precautions:

1. Never swim alone or unobserved.

2. Swim only in supervised areas.

3. Watch children and friends while they are swimming. You may notice a dangerous situation before a lifeguard does.

4. Follow the safety rules at the place you swim.

5. Do not attempt to swim long distances or a long way from shore if you are not in excellent physical condition or if you are tired.

(continued on p. 81)

Did You Know That . . .

Not only does survival floating conserve energy, but it also conserves body heat: swimming or treading water cools the body 35 percent faster.

It's the dead of summer, and the battle to stay cool can't be won with an iced-tea break. Your friend Bob, who has just filled his new in-ground pool with water, wants to celebrate summer by having you and a few other close friends over for a pool party. You get to Bob's, and before you know it you're relaxing on a lounge chair. Bob has the barbecue going. He serves you a couple of burgers, which you wash down with a beer or two. Now you're really feeling good, except for the heat. But today, beating the heat doesn't pose a problem. As you walk over to the pool ladder to take a dip, Bob challenges you to a race. You never learned how to dive, but how hard can it be? Ready . . . set . . . Stop!

Jumping in Feet First

For too many people, this typical pool-party scene illustrates where their problems began. More than 800 Americans each year suffer spinal cord injuries as a result of diving accidents, according to the National Spinal Cord Injury Data Research Center. The result is quadriplegia or paraplegia in about 95 percent of these incidences—a frighteningly high number by any measure.

A revealing portrait of those who most often sustain spinal injuries from diving into a swimming pool has been drawn by researchers M. Alexander Gabrielsen, Ph.D., and Mary Spivey of Nova University in Fort Lauderdale FL, who studied 340 such cases.

Almost invariably, the victims were males between the ages of 18 and 31 who had no formal diving training. The accident occurred on the first dive of their first visit to a pool. They had no knowledge that diving in a pool could end in a broken neck, permanent paralysis and even death. Add to this the alcohol drinking that often goes on at poolside, along with the "horseplay" young men enjoy taking part in, and you have the makings for a catastrophe.

The same study gives a clear picture of the type of environment in which diving accidents most frequently occur. More than half of the injuries take place in a pool located at a private home, with the remaining accidents taking place at an apartment house complex, hotel or motel pool. Like the accident victim, the pool operator is not aware of the dangers that can result from diving into a swimming pool. There are no depth markings on or in the pool, nor are there warning signs prohibiting diving. This is particularly significant, because seven out of eight diving disasters are sustained by victims who struck bottom where the water was less than five-feet deep.

Each year, some 100,000 people receive medical or surgical treatment due to diving accidents. The great tragedy is that virtually all of these accidents could have been avoided if proper precautions had been taken. This includes, according to researchers, diving-related spinal cord injuries. Some studies have also noted that a significant number of those who have drowned because of spinal cord injuries could have been saved . . . if only those at the pool had immediately taken note that an accident had occurred and were capable of providing prompt and proper rescue procedures.

Unfortunately, "if onlys" do not restore life or limb function. Investigators Gabrielsen and Spivey, however, offer a simple and effective four-pronged plan of action that would substantially reduce the number of diving accidents that occur each year: Educate people about the dangers of diving into a pool. Communicate at the pool site by using clearly visible water-depth markers and signs posting pool rules. Regulate the design, construction, operation and maintenance of swimming pools. And finally, learn more about diving accidents and how to provide more effective medical treatment to the injured.

NOTE: Feet First First Time is a program that was developed in Florida to help educate children about diving and water safety. For more information, contact: Feet First First Time, Inc., West Florida Regional Medical Center, Pensacola FL, or call 904/478–4460, extension 4837.

Source: Eric Mood, *Priorities* (Summer 1989), p. 35.

Take Steps to Avoid Childhood Drownings

Soon after becoming a commissioner at the Consumer Product Safety Commission (CPSC) in 1984, I became very interested in the problem of childhood drowning, which claimed the lives of an estimated 236 children under five years of age in 1985. In several states, including California and Arizona, it has been the leading cause of accidental death in the home for children under five.

Childhood drowning is hardly an issue that elicits a lukewarm response. A recent incident in California illustrates that point and is worth relating because it depicts an all-too-common scenario. The incident took place in the afternoon. The mother of a two-year old was in the laundry room. Her little boy was by her side but disappeared suddenly. When she couldn't locate him, she called the police. She feared that he had fallen into the backyard swimming pool. The pool had been neglected and, consequently, was darkened by algae, making it impossible to determine visually whether the boy had, in fact, fallen into the pool.

Hopes of finding her son at a neighbor's were shattered when rescue workers recovered his limp body from the pool. This mother's nightmare became a reality. It was initially reported that the boy was in a deep coma, showing signs of severe brain injury. Today, he is confined to Agnew State Hospital in California with severe brain damage. He will not recover. . . .

This is not just an emotional issue. Even people who take the purely economic view are staggered by the consequences of these accidents. Some severely brain-damaged children have initial hospital stays in excess of 120 days, costing more than $150,000. After initial stays, caring for these children costs an average of $90,000 for their 12 to 18 month post-accident lifespan. In both human and economic terms, there are no skeptics when it comes to the necessity, and the urgency, of stopping this national heartbreak.

Over the last several years some significant steps have been taken by the CPSC to learn as much as possible about circumstances surrounding drownings of children under five in residential swimming pools. This has helped us determine how much of the problem is preventable and what steps can be taken to reduce child drownings.

The Circumstances

During the summer of 1986, the CPSC conducted a study of drowning and near-drowning incidents involving children under five. The study was conducted in eight counties in the states of Arizona, California, and Florida. A case-reporting network of coroners, medical examiners, emergency medical service personnel, fire and police, hospital staff, trauma registries, and public health officials was established. One hundred forty-two incidents were reported, including 40 deaths.

The goal of the study was to identify the circumstances surrounding the accidental drowning of children in backyard swimming pools, and from that information to develop and implement plans for reducing the risk of drowning.

The analysis of the study showed that victims at risk are under five years of age—particularly one to two year olds. Males are more often involved, which is not surprising because child development literature shows males to be more physically active, and they are prone to do more outdoor exploring at this age. Young children, especially those exposed to swimming pools, expect to have fun in the water. Bathtime is playtime. Almost all victims were exposed to the pools in the context of fun and play and were attracted to the water rather than fearful. This indicates that children may not perceive a risk associated with going into a pool and cannot be relied upon to follow rules.

Looking at the social and physical environments enables us to determine how the child got into the pool. In general, accident investigations indicate that conscientious parents, who understand the need for supervision, experienced a short *lapse* in supervision, not necessarily a *lack* of supervision. In almost half of the cases, the child was last seen in the house. Parents perceive the house as a "safe area" for children. In the drowning cases, however, it appears that house doors leading to the pool area were the weak link. Even children between one and two have been found to unlock and open both hinged and sliding glass doors.

The study showed that when there was a fence between the house and the pool, some children were still able to reach the pool because the gate was left open or because the gate latch or fence needed repair. However, the fence and gate that separate the house from the pool should serve as a more effective barrier than a house door. More than one level of protection has the potential for preventing and delaying access to the pool. Those vital few minutes when a lapse does occur can be bought by having more than one level of protection between the child and the pool.

An analysis of the accidents themselves shows that they were: 1) silent and 2) preventable. Normally children cry out if they are in trouble. The silent nature of a child drowning distinguishes it from other hazards because of its inability to overcome lapses in parental supervision. In three-fourths of the cases for which information is available, the child was estimated to have been missing for five minutes or less. Following the accidents, the parents indicated that they were aware of the danger of drowning before the accident occurred, but expressed surprise at just how easily and rapidly an accident could occur.

This study shows that we are not up against one large threat—a Goliath we might bring down with a single blow or a series of regulations—but many small hazards, any one of which can lead to death or serious injury: unlocked doors, broken locks, an attractive ball left floating in a pool, a telephone call at an inopportune moment.

Measures to Take

As I have said, distractions, even of the most ordinary sort, can lead to death or serious injury.

There are measures parents can take to supplement supervision:

* A fence on all four sides of the pool (separating the pool from the house and from the yard area) with a properly secured gate can provide a second level of protection. The fence should be at least five feet high with vertical spacing of no more than four inches.
* Access through house doors could be reduced if all doors leading from the house directly to the pool area were secured with a supplemental latch at a height of at least five feet. Screen doors should also have a supplemental latch at this same height.
* Floating objects should be removed from the pool when the pool is not in use because they may be seen as toys by young children who may be attracted to them.
* Emergency care could be administered in the event of a submersion accident if all adult family members and child caretakers, in homes with swimming pools and where there are children under five years of age, learned CPR.

Another story helps to illustrate this last point. Recently in Orange County, Calif., two toddlers—21 months and 18 months—nearly drowned in a backyard spa. The mother, a former nurse, stepped into another room across the hall to change clothes. In the less than five minutes she was gone, the pair toddled from their playroom and somehow got past a sliding screen door to the backyard. When the mother didn't hear their voices, she went looking and called for them on the patio. Then she saw "Molly" floating on her back in the spa. "Kathleen" was on the bottom. She jumped in, pulled them out and began CPR on both of them—giving chest compressions on one, while blowing breath into the other. They were taking their first breaths on their own by the time paramedics arrived. This mother's training in CPR gave her the ability to save these two little ones. CPR is something everyone, especially parents, should know how to administer. . . .

Source: Carol Dawson, *Consumer's Research* (July 1988), pp. 26–28.

6. Alcohol and swimming do not mix. Avoid alcohol and all other forms of psychoactive drugs if you plan to go near the water.

In addition, it is important to avoid diving accidents, which injure more than 100,000 Americans each year. For further information, see the box entitled "Jumping in Feet First."

Boating

Like swimming, boating should be approached enthusiastically but with caution. A boating accident can turn a happy day on a boat into a devastating, even deadly, experience.

Capsizing About half of all boating accidents involve capsizing, which is most frequently caused by overloading. To reduce the risk of capsizing, the number of passengers must not exceed the boat's capacity. Many boaters believe the number of seats in

Did You Know That . . .

One of the major dangers in many boating accidents is hypothermia. Cold water saps body heat far more rapidly than cold air. A person of average body size will remain conscious for no more than 2 to 3 hours in 50-degree water and one half hour or less in 40-degree water.

FIGURE 4.2
Capsizing

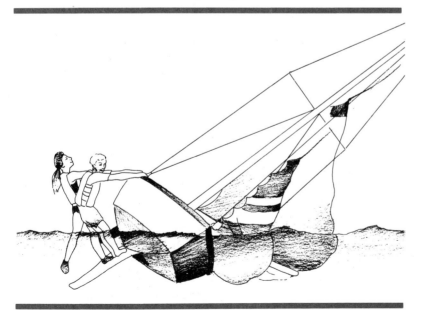

If your boat does capsize, stay with the boat. In some instances it may be possible to right a capsized boat by standing on the centerboard and applying leverage.

the boat indicates the proper number of passengers, but that is not always the case. A better way to determine the correct number is to multiply the boat's length by its width and then divide that figure by 15. The weight capacity of many new boats is indicated on the craft.

Always bear in mind the risk of capsizing while boating. When boarding a boat or changing positions, keep low and step in the center of the craft. Never stand up in a small boat once the craft is in motion.

If a boat does capsize because of a storm or other accident, stay with the boat. A capsized boat often stays afloat indefinitely—especially newer ones, which often have extra flotation built into them. Hanging on and waiting for help is almost always the safest move. Trying to swim ashore, on the other hand, is a mistake. The distance is usually further than it looks and even an excellent swimmer may have trouble getting there.

Operating Practices   Boating accidents can also result from unsafe operating practices, such as speeding, failing to observe the right of way, or cutting in front of other craft. The best way to ensure safety is to observe a set of official boating regulations called "The Rules of the Road." There are separate sets of rules for sailboats and power boats. Among the rules for safe powerboating are the following:

1. *Approaching Situation:* When two power boats meet head-on, each should keep to the starboard (right), allowing the other vessel to pass to the port (left) side.

2. *Crossing Situation:* When two power boats approach each other at right angles, the boat on the right has the right of way.

3. *Overtaking Situation:* When a power boat overtakes another boat, the faster boat may pass, provided that there is enough room. In this situation, the craft being overtaken has the right of way.

4. *Nonmotor Craft:* Sailboats, rowboats, canoes, and other non-motor craft have the right of way in meeting and crossing situations with power boats.

Storms   Even an experienced boater must pay attention to weather and wind conditions. As a preventive measure, listen to a marine weather forecast before leaving and be prepared to adjust your plans or postpone your trip if hazardous weather is antici-

FIGURE 4.3
"Rules of the Road" for Power Boats

Meeting

When 2 boats are on courses that will result in their meeting head on or nearly so, each should steer to the right.

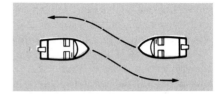

Crossing

When crossing, the boat on the right is the "privileged" boat and has the right of way. The boat on the left is the "burdened" vessel and should slow down or change course as necessary so as to pass astern of the other boat.

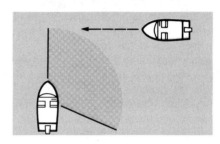

Passing

When one boat is overtaking another, the boat being overtaken (passed) is the "privileged" vessel. Provided there is adequate room, the faster boat may pass on either side while staying clear of the slower vessel.

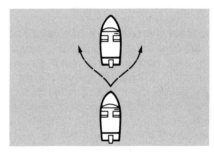

The situations described above are based on the United States Coast Guard rules for inland navigation. Operating rules for rivers, lakes, and international waters are similar, but boaters should always follow the specific rules for the area in which they are operating.

pated. Once under way, you should make a point of periodically monitoring the marine radio for weather updates and small craft warnings. You should also be on the alert for any signs of an impending storm. These include a darkening sky, thunder, lightning, radio static, and cool wind blasts. Because it is always more prudent to avoid storms than to weather them at sea, plan to seek a safe port immediately whenever small craft warnings are issued or signs of a storm appear.

(continued on p. 86)

Better Safe

Boats are safe, but people aren't.

• You've hooked into a big bass as you drift along in the river current, and you're not going to let this one get away. Your friend is leaning way out, ready to net the fish, but as it sees the boat it flips away with a splash. Your fishing buddy scoops far out with the net and suddenly tumbles in. You wait for him to come up, see him momentarily downriver as he struggles to the surface, and then watch him disappear again as you try to start the motor to get down to him.

• From where you're anchored behind the point, dusk comes slowly after sunset across the lake, and in the distance you can hear a runabout racing along the shore beyond. Suddenly, it comes around the point, heading straight for you at its normal speed—full throttle—and you can see two kids sitting on the gunnels. When the driver spots you, he swings hard over, and his boat flips as it smashes into your stern. The three kids are thrown into the water, and the runabout rights itself and, with the motor still running, heads off in a long arc toward the shore. For hours, you paddle in a circle in the dark but can locate only one of the youngsters. None wore life jackets.

• An elderly friend rents a skiff to head up a tidewater bay where you've recommended the fishing. The dockmaster remembers laughing when he showed up with his favorite tackle in one hand and his favorite bottle in the other. He hadn't wanted the big, powerful outboard—just a little rowboat with a kicker, bait bucket and ice chest. When he doesn't get back at sundown, they find the skiff floating out on the ebb tide, empty. There's no way to know whether he had a heart attack, slipped when he was casting, or stood up to relieve himself and fell in—as often happens, he may have cramped up in the cold water due to hypothermia and, because he wasn't a good swimmer, couldn't pull himself back up aboard; or perhaps he tried to swim for shore.

• Late-afternoon thunderheads are piling up, and there have been forecasts of a possible summer squall line powering through before sunset. The sky has turned dark along the horizon, but it's hard to tell which way the storm is traveling because right now there is no wind and the water is calm. Out on the horizon, silhouetted against the dark clouds, there is a fishing skiff, and you can see someone standing up, pulling the starter cord over and over. He's probably been running from place to place all day and never checked his gas tank. But now, he disappears in sheets of rain as the wind comes, and you head back to port. In less than an hour, when the storm has blown through and the sky clears, you look back out but the boat is gone. Later, when it's found floating and full of water but fisherman and tackle are gone, it is apparent that the waves must have rolled aboard and swamped the boat so that it capsized and dumped everything overboard before righting itself. As in so many cases, no one will know just what happened.

Statistics covering boating accidents are very incomplete. The Coast Guard estimates that it receives information on only 5 to 10 percent of all accidents, even though the law states: "The operator of a vessel used for recreational purposes is required to file a report in writing whenever an accident results in loss of life or disappearance from a vessel; an injury that requires medical treatment beyond first aid; or property damage in excess of $200 or complete loss of vessel. Reports in death and injury cases must be submitted within 48 hours. Reports in other cases must be submitted within 10 days. Reports must be submitted to the reporting authority in the state where the accident occurred." The Coast Guard has a form to assist the operator in filing the required written report.

Most boating-related deaths are reported one way or another, and though the majority of other accidents on the water are not, it's still easy to look back over the years of records and see what the causes are—and how to avoid them. Fortunately for us, we go boating for the fun of it.

There is no excuse for heading out with inadequate skill and equipment in bad weather or into conditions and places that we haven't studied in advance.

It's been estimated that 90 percent of the 70 million of us who go boating (and who spend $17 billion a year to do it) have had little or no boating education, little boating experience, and may consider ourselves fishermen, sportsmen or water-skiers rather than boatmen. Statistics indicate that more than half of all boating accidents are the fault of an operator who may have been under the influence of alcohol, drugs or both.

The Coast Guard has found a dozen types of accidents that can result in damage or fatalities. Their order of frequency in 1986 . . . was as follows: collision with another vessel; collision with a fixed object; capsizing; falls overboard; fire or explosion from fuel; grounding; swamping or flooding; collision with a floating object; sinking; being struck by a boat or propeller; and fire or explosion from causes other than fuel. Two additional categories were "other" and that unfortunate "unknown." Accidents involving a collision with another vessel were 10 times more prevalent than those in the second most frequent category, collisions with a fixed object. Most fatalities were the result of capsizing; falls overboard were second.

The cause of the largest number of accidents was given as that old favorite, "other vessel at fault." The second most frequent category, however, was "inattention or carelessness," and the third was "improper lookout." The cause of most fatalities was "unknown," but "strong current and rough waters" came in second, and "inattention and carelessness" was third. Other causes for both accidents and deaths included overloading; improper weight distribution; sitting on gunnels/transom/bow or back of seat; movement of passengers; anchoring; leaning overboard; water entering boat; problems with fuel, electrical, power or heat equipment; problems with steering or throttle controls; improper navigation lights; or starting in gear. Accidents also occurred because of high-speed maneuvering and acceleration; obstructed view; violations of rules of the road; speeding; navigational errors; wake

or wave striking the boat; strong current; rough waters; slippery surface or deck; poor visibility; submerged objects; and ignition of spilled fuel. They all sound familiar.

Steering and throttle-problem accidents were far down on the list, though they are sometimes a cop-out for boatmen who want to blame "mechanical failure" instead of driver stupidity. Unfortunately, afloat as well as ashore, the great American tradition of "When at fault, sue someone else" still takes place. The listed causes of accidents are determined by studies of the accident reports, incidentally, rather than from operator claims. Obviously, careless operation cannot be blamed on the boat.

The largest number of fatalities on the water in 1986 were recorded as "cause unknown." Next comes strong current or rough waters, followed by inattention or carelessness, overloading, improper weight distribution, speeding, improper lookout, and leaning over the edge of the boat. Most accidents occurred on a calm, sunny day during a summer afternoon on a lake, pond, reservoir or gravel pit while cruising or drift fishing, and though they usually happen in an open outboard (because there are more of them in use on the water), by far the most accidents take place with boats of 16 to 26 feet, though most deaths occur with craft of less than 16 feet in length.

The boat driver was usually between 26 and 50 years old, with the next most dangerous age category being those drivers older than 50. He had more than 500 hours of boating experience but no formal instruction. Two people were on board in the case of most accidents, but only one was in the boat when most fatalities happened. In most cases of accidents and deaths, approved life preservers were aboard and accessible but not used.

These statistics provide clear pictures of how, when and where accidents happen, but less-than-full answers for how to prevent them. Any accident or death on the water is one too many, but there are differences of opinion about the best cures. The state of Maryland recently passed a requirement for mandatory boating education, and the law may become a model for other states as well. Few boatmen want more laws—who does?—but many are willing to see legislation that controls ignorant skippers who overload, overpower, overspeed, endanger other craft with oversize wakes, or just fall overboard from overconfidence. And unlike a car, with a boat or plane it's inconvenient to try to stop, get out and walk home.

One recent survey of experienced boatmen indicated that a majority favor driver's licenses for skippers. This is a solution that seems to have frightened boat builders, dealers and rental operators for many years. Apparently, the only thing that worries them more than having customers drown is to have customers discouraged from buying. Why get into the charges, red tape and bureaucracy of boat driving licenses, it's argued, when automotive driver tests and licenses haven't cured car accidents? True enough. But does that mean licenses for driving cars, or aircraft, should be abandoned?

Statistics do show that the ratio of the number of fatalities to the growing number of boats in use is going down every year, so boating must be getting safer. But the thousands of people who are killed or injured annually plus the $20 million in damages, as determined from the small percentage of accidents reported, stay about the same and indicate that we have a lot of improving to do. Questionnaires show that boatmen say they are very concerned about safety and want to learn more about it. Readership surveys show that it may be approximately the last thing people are willing to read about. So, if you've gotten this far, congratulations. Enjoying our sport by picking the right boat, and learning how and when and where to use it to stay alive, is worth some thought.

Source: Bill McKeown, *Outdoor Life* (September 1988), p. 58, 60–61.

If caught in a sudden squall, every person in the boat should put on a **personal flotation device** (life jacket) immediately. If you are on a sailing vessel, the sails should be taken down as quickly as possible. If you are in a small boat, sit on the floorboards to lower the boat's center of gravity. This will also reduce wind resistance and make the boat easier to control. The best way to navigate rough seas is to meet the waves at a slight angle rather than head-on.

Fires and Explosions Small power craft are usually fueled with gasoline, which can be extremely dangerous when not handled properly. A cup of gasoline spilled in the **bilge** has the potential explosive power of 15 sticks of dynamite. Because there are many ignition sources in and around the engine compartment, the following safety precautions should be observed when handling boat fuels:

Personal flotation device: A life belt, life preserver, or other device designed to help an individual keep afloat in the water.

Bilge: The lowest portion of the interior space enclosed within the hull of a boat or other such vessel.

1. Avoid fueling at night.

2. Stop all engines and motors while fueling.

3. Do not smoke, strike matches, or throw switches.

4. Make sure the boat is moored securely.

5. After fueling, wipe up all spilled fuel and run the boat ventilation system (the blower) before starting the engine.

6. Do not fill portable tanks while on the boat.

The pleasures of boating can be great. Careful and safe boat handling can keep those pleasures from turning into tragedy.

RECREATIONAL VEHICLE SAFETY

During the last decade, sales of all-terrain vehicles (ATVs) boomed. By 1989 there were an estimated 5 million ATV riders in the country. Unfortunately, accidents have also increased. More than 600 people have died and 275,000 have been injured in ATV mishaps. Nearly half the deaths and injuries involved youngsters under the age of 16.

FIGURE 4.4
All-Terrain Vehicle

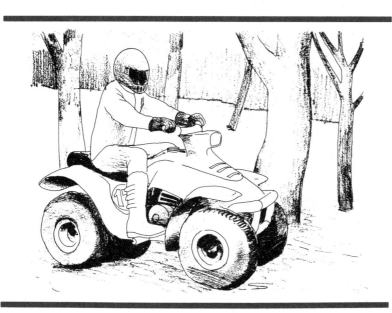

An all-terrain vehicle (ATV) is designed for off-the-road use only and should not be ridden on pavement. When riding an ATV, it is important to wear protective clothing, respect the environment and all local rules, and never carry passengers.

The ATVenturer's Pledge

I will learn all the mechanical controls and safety devices of my ATV and check them each time before I ride.

I will wear a helmet at all times and other protective clothing suitable to the environment when I ride.

I will ask an instructor or qualified rider to teach me proper riding skills and I will practice until my skills are well developed before entering an unfamiliar area.

I will respect the laws when I ride and I will honor the rules where I ride.

I will not carry passengers on my ATV.

I will be courteous to other riders and persons by offering right-of way and respecting areas that are posted closed.

I will not use alcohol or other drugs when I ride.

I will not litter the area nor damage plant life where I ride.

I will only lend my ATV to someone I have personally instructed in its safe and appropriate use.

I have made this pledge because I am a thoughtful ATV rider. I accept my responsibility for preserving the sport, and the safety of its enthusiasts. And . . . I want everyone to have fun with the great ATVenture.

My name is _____

Source: Specialty Vehicle Institute of America, Costa Mesa, CA.

One attitude that leads to ATV accidents is the belief that an ATV is a toy rather than a vehicle. In fact, ATVs are specialized vehicles that require specific skills that are different from those used for motorcycles, bicycles, or automobiles. Learning those skills and following safe operating rules are essential to safe riding.

If you are interested in driving an ATV, take an accredited course in ATV operations. [1] Always wear proper clothing, including helmet, boots, gloves, eye protection, and a long-sleeved jacket or top. As with all motor vehicles, do not drive an ATV if you are under the influence of alcohol or another psychoactive drug. Finally, do not carry passengers; ATVs are designed for one passenger (the driver) only.

HUNTING SAFETY

Hunting attracts an enthusiastic following. Because of the inherent dangers of the sport, knowing and attending to all safety precautions is necessary to ensure safety.

Approximately 60 percent of gun casualties involve individuals under the age of 21. Many states require people under 16 to complete a hunter safety course before being allowed to hunt with a gun or bow. [2]

A hunter must be sure that he or she is clearly visible to other hunters and cannot be mistaken for game. Studies show that hunter orange is the most effective color. It is bright and fluorescent and is more visible at dusk or dawn than other colors.

Accidents and injuries with firearms are often caused by poor safety habits and ignorance. Every hunter should memorize and practice "The Ten Commandants of Firearm Safety." [3]

1. Treat every gun as though it were loaded—whether or not it is.

2. Keep the **muzzle** under control, so that even if you trip and fall the muzzle is not pointing at yourself or anyone else.

3. Be sure the barrel and action are clear of obstructions and use only the proper ammunition for the gun.

4. Be sure of the target before pulling the trigger.

5. Unload all guns not in use.

6. Do not play around with a gun.

7. Avoid climbing trees, fences, or other objects when carrying a gun.

8. Make sure there is a solid backstop for target practice.

9. Store guns and ammunition separately; keep both out of the reach of children.

10. Never use a gun when under the influence of alcohol or other psychoactive drugs.

Did You Know That . . .

From 1963 to 1973, 84,633 people in the United States died of gunshot wounds. Only about half that number—46,752—were killed during those same years in the Vietnam War.

Muzzle: The mouth or opening of the barrel of a gun.

WILDERNESS SURVIVAL

Today, outdoor enthusiasts can go into wilderness areas with little difficulty on snowmobiles, ATVs, and trail bikes. Unfortunately, getting in is sometimes easier than getting out. People can become accidentally stranded when vehicles break down or the trail is lost. As a result, survival in the wilderness has become an important safety technique.

The first step to wilderness survival is to avoid getting lost in the first place by following these guidelines:

1. Always let someone know where you are going and when you will be back. Leave your car license and other information with friends.

2. Always carry area maps.

3. Avoid going alone. Use the buddy system.

4. Be prepared. Take enough lightweight, high-energy food to last a few days.

5. Carry the proper survival equipment, including a knife, waterproof matches in a container, a candle, a canteen of water, and fire-starting materials.

6. Plan your trip so that you get back to camp before dark. Take note of landmarks during the day to help you return to base camp. Check your map and your compass periodically throughout the day.

Hypothermia

Phoebe and Kevin had no idea it would be so windy in the wilderness. They had set out for a day of hiking and a night of camping and because it was early spring, they did not dress warmly. Toward evening there was a dramatic change in the weather. A strong northwesterly wind arose, the temperature fell sharply, and a light rain began to fall. Phoebe grew tired. Noticing how pale she looked, Kevin suggested she rest while he finished pitching camp. Soon Phoebe began shivering uncontrollably; concerned, Kevin hurriedly helped Phoebe remove her wet clothes and put on a dry shirt and sweater. When her shivering did not subside, Kevin warmed some rocks in the fire and placed them under her armpits. He was able to carry her into the warm interior of their tent, where they spent the night.

Phoebe was suffering from **hypothermia**, a condition in which the temperature of the inner core of the body drops below the normal body temperature of 98.6 degrees Fahrenheit. When hypothermia occurs, the body loses heat faster than it can produce it. Without treatment it can result in death.

Because hypothermia has few symptoms, it sometimes goes undetected during early stages. There are some early signs of which to be aware, such as uncontrollable shivering, cold, pale skin, and general **apathy**.

As the temperature of the inner core decreases further, the sufferer may become disoriented and may exhibit muscle rigidity, slurred speech, and a slowed pulse and respiration rate. If left untreated, he or she can lapse into a **coma** and suffer cardiac arrest.

Hypothermia is caused by a combination of cold air, wetness, and windchill. The cold air itself does not have to be extreme. People can die from hypothermia in temperatures well above freezing if they are wet or the wind is stiff. A slight breeze will carry heat away from bare skin much more quickly than still air. Windchill combined with wetness will extract heat from the body very quickly.

The first thing to do for someone suffering from hypothermia is to reduce heat loss by getting him or her out of the wind, removing wet clothing, and replacing it with dry clothing or blankets or both. Then apply external heat to the sides of the chest, neck, armpits, and groin area. Use any available heat source; heated rocks wrapped in towels will do if nothing else is available. Be careful not to burn the victim and do not give him or her alcohol or coffee; hot beverages have little benefit and alcohol is harmful. If the victim must be moved, transport him or her gently in a lying-down position with the head lower than the feet.

The best way to prevent hypothermia is to reduce or avoid exposure to cold and wet elements. Wear proper clothing, use proper cold-weather equipment, and set up camp thoroughly and completely before exhaustion sets in. Moreover, be prepared for cold weather or a sudden storm, regardless of season. Weather can change rapidly, particularly in mountainous regions where sudden storms can cause hypothermia even during the summer. Always bring extra sweaters and dry clothing on camping trips, just in case.

Frostbite
Cold weather can also cause **frostbite**, which can in turn lead to serious injury. Frostbite occurs when body cells or tissues freeze.

Hypothermia: A condition characterized by a subnormal body temperature, accompanied by drowsiness and significantly reduced respiratory and heart rates. Hypothermia is a medical emergency and can lead to coma and death if left untreated.

Apathy: A lack of feeling or emotion.

Coma: A state of unconsciousness and unresponsiveness characterized by an inability to respond to outside stimuli.

Frostbite: Damage to tissues caused by exposure to extremely cold conditions; symptoms include numbness and discoloration. It can lead to a serious infection, such as gangrene, if left untreated.

FIGURE 4.5
First Aid for Frostbite

Frostbite is damage to tissues caused by below-freezing temperatures. Frostbite and hypothermia often develop at the same time. Hypothermia must be treated first. Prompt treatment for frostbite is essential to minimize the long-term effects. In the following order, here's what to do:

DO
- Seek shelter and expose the frostbitten area. Remove clothing and items (jewelry or watch) that constrict circulation.
- Warm up the affected area by covering it gently with warm hands or clothing. Or warm frostbitten hands in the victim's armpits. Warm feet in a companion's armpits.
- Dip the affected area in warm water (less than 110° F), if available. Cover with a sterile dressing.

DON'T rub frostbitten areas.
DON'T apply direct heat to the affected area.
DON'T try to burst blisters.
DON'T permit the victim to walk on a frostbitten foot.

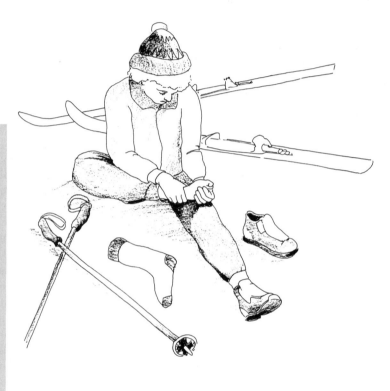

Treat frostbite by warming affected areas with warm hands, clothing, or other warm parts of the body, such as the armpits.

Blood vessels: Any of the structures that transport blood throughout the body; the arteries, veins, and capillaries.

Left untreated, the condition can lead to tissue death and permanent loss of function.

Frostbite occurs in extremely cold conditions, when the body protects itself by constricting surface **blood vessels** in an attempt to keep warm the larger supply of blood in the core of the inner body. When this happens, the hands and feet cool very quickly.

The extent of frostbite injury depends upon the outside temperature, wind velocity, wetness, and type of clothing. Stress, fatigue, smoking, and drinking alcohol can worsen the condition.

Frostbite is usually classified as either superficial or deep. Superficial frostbite involves injury to the fingers, ears, nose, and cheeks. Symptoms include white or grayish-yellow skin color and pain occurring early but subsiding with numbness. Deep frostbite usually involves hands and feet. The affected tissues will feel cold, solid, hard, and numb. Blisters may appear in 12 to 36 hours.

The best treatment for superficial frostbite is to submerge the stricken area in water at a temperature between 102 and 105 degrees Fahrenheit. Do not rub the area.

No frostbite victim should ever be permitted to walk on thawed toes or feet. This could result in serious additional damage. Frozen feet should not be thawed unless the victim can be transported without walking. Do not rewarm an area if you cannot protect it from refreezing. This can cause more damage than the original frostbite. Victims of deep frostbite require immediate medical attention.

Americans spend thousands of hours every year enjoying outdoor recreation—swimming, boating, riding recreational vehicles, and hiking in the wilderness. These leisure-time activities can provide well-earned rest and relaxation and can be completely safe if participants remember to observe the basic rules of accident prevention. 🅦

Did You Know That . . .

To avoid slipping on ice, tilt your body forward, take short steps, and set your feet down flat. To reduce injury if you do fall, go limp and try to roll as you land.

Fires and Occupational Safety

EVER SINCE its discovery in prehistoric times, fire has been indispensable to human society. Some form of fire heats our homes, cooks our food, powers our businesses, and often produces electricity. Yet as helpful as fire is, it can be deadly when uncontrolled.

The United States has the highest per capita fire death rate of any country in the industrialized world. In 1988 there were an estimated 2,436,550 fires in this country, resulting in 6,215 deaths and more than 200,000 injuries. More than 74 percent of all structural fires and 80 percent of the fatalities occurred on residential properties. Property losses were estimated at more than 8 billion dollars. [1]

FIRE CHEMISTRY

In order for fire to occur, 3 basic elements must be present: fuel, heat, and oxygen. These 3 elements combine to cause **combustion**.

Fuel

Combustible substances, or fuels, are of 3 types: (1) solids such as wood, paper, cloth, and some forms of plastic; (2) liquids such as gasoline, alcohol, oil, and kerosene; and (3) gases such as **acetylene**, **propane**, and **hydrogen**. Of these 3, **flammable** liquids are the most hazardous and the most unpredictable.

Heat

Heat is necessary to initiate combustion. When fuel becomes hot enough, it begins to **vaporize**. When the vapors mix with oxygen, the result is a chemical reaction that releases heat, flame, and

Combustion: A chemical process characterized by the rapid oxidation of one or more combustible substances (fuel) accompanied by the generation of heat and light; the burning process.

Acetylene: A colorless gas used chiefly as a fuel for high temperature torches used to cut or weld heavy metals.

Propane: A highly flammable gas primarily obtained from natural gas or refined from petroleum; used chiefly as a fuel.

Hydrogen: An abundant gaseous nonmetallic element (symbol H) that is the lightest and simplest gas; it is highly flammable.

Flammable: Capable of being easily ignited or set on fire.

Vaporize: To change from a liquid or a solid to a gas.

smoke. Fuel must be heated to its kindling temperature in order to ignite.

Oxygen

As mentioned above, vapors must combine with oxygen for combustion to occur. Fire consumes oxygen and turns it into carbon dioxide. Because fire is so dependent on it, cutting off the oxygen supply to a flame will extinguish a fire instantly.

FIRE PREVENTION IN THE HOME

Statistics show that more than 80 percent of fatal fires start in the living room, bedroom, or kitchen. [2] A few basic safety measures in these areas can provide protection.

Kitchen: The stove top, oven, toaster oven, and broiler are all heat sources that can start fires. Towels, curtains, and paper products, as well as loose-fitting or flowing garments, should be kept away from them.

Grease fires can occur during cooking and should be extinguished by placing a lid on the pan or by turning off the burner and applying baking soda to the flames. Do not use water: The oxygen it contains will spread the fire.

Living Room and Bedroom: Cigarettes and electricity are the 2 most common causes of fire in these areas. Provide large ashtrays for smokers and dispose of cigarette butts and ashes properly. Do not overload electrical circuits or use cheap extension cords to power appliances such as irons and heaters that require large amounts of electricity.

Wood-burning Stoves and Fireplaces: Sparks and hot coals from wood-burning stoves and fireplaces can ignite rugs and furnishings. Using a screen in front of an open fire will keep sparks from reaching flammables. Because stoves can become red hot, it is possible for them to ignite combustibles, such as curtains or even walls and floors. A freestanding stove, therefore, should be installed by a professional on a fireproof base and away from unprotected walls.

Wood stoves can also cause chimney fires, which occur when **creosote** builds up in the chimney and is ignited by a spark. Creosote burns at a very high temperature, and if there are cracks in the flue the fire can spread to rafters, beams, or the roof. No matter how careful you are, creosote will eventually collect inside your chimney. Check the chimney periodically; more than 1/4 inch of crusty, flaky, or powdery deposit requires a thorough cleaning by a professional chimney sweep. A tar-like, gummy, or

Did You Know That . . .

It is estimated that up to one-half of all residential fires are caused by cigarettes.

Creosote: A combustible, hard, black, lacquer-like deposit consisting of incompletely burned combustion byproducts that tends to accumulate on the interior of wood-burning stoves and flues; if allowed to build up to dangerous levels, it represents a serious fire hazard.

FIGURE 5.1
Wood Stove Safety

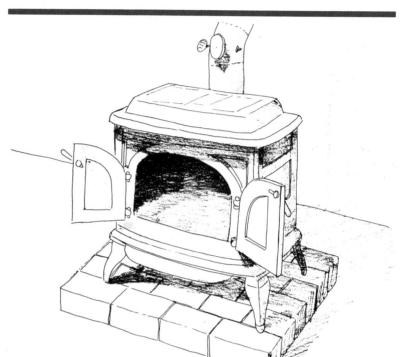

Regular cleaning of a wood-burning stove, flue, and chimney is essential to help prevent chimney fires. The buildup of creosote, the main source of chimney fires, can be reduced by using only well-seasoned, dry wood.

hard-glazed substance coating the chimney indicates that the system is not functioning properly and should be checked by a professional immediately. [3]

Electrical Fires: Electrical wiring in the home is usually protected from overheating by circuit breakers or fuses. However, these safety devices may not always afford the protection needed from an overloaded extension cord or a faulty appliance. The following tips can help prevent electrical fires:

1. Do not overload circuits. Frequent activation of fuses and circuit breakers is an indication that an overload is present,

usually in the form of too many appliances on the same circuit or a malfunctioning appliance.

2. Do not tamper with the circuit breakers or fuses in an effort to keep them from blowing.

3. Use only the proper extension cords for specific jobs. Light duty cords should not be used with appliances. Never use cords that are cracked or frayed.

4. Do not route an electrical cord over nails or hooks or under carpets. This can damage the cord's insulation.

5. Keep heaters and other appliances away from flammable materials. Even light bulbs can ignite paper or lightweight cloth.

Flammable Liquid Fires: Many liquids used around the house are flammable. Using or storing them improperly can cause a disaster. Store all turpentine, varnish, kerosene, and alcohol in a well-ventilated area far away from ignition or heat sources.

Gasoline is the most commonly used flammable liquid and possibly the most dangerous. It has a **flash point** of −45 degrees Fahrenheit, which means that it will ignite instantaneously in the presence of a flame at any temperature down to this level. It should be stored in an approved safety can that is specifically constructed for flammable liquids with vents and with flame-arresting screens in the filling and dispensing spouts. Store only the amount that you need.

Spontaneous Combustion: **Spontaneous combustion** occurs when the temperature of a material increases without drawing heat from its surroundings. Rubbish piles, boxes of old clothes, dust rags, oily rags, or paint rags can all be sources of such fires. These materials should be stored in metal, airtight containers.

SMOKE ALARMS

Unfortunately, not all fires can be prevented. Despite careful measures fires can still occur; when they do, often the only thing protecting a family from tragedy is a smoke alarm system. Properly installed and maintained **smoke detectors** save thousands of lives every year.

Installation
Smoke detectors should be installed on every level of a home. At the very least, a detector should be placed outside each of the

Flash point: The lowest temperature at which a flammable liquid gives off a quantity of vapor sufficient to produce combustion if exposed to an open flame.

Spontaneous combustion: Combustion that occurs without the introduction of an external flame or heat source, usually as the result of the decomposition of organic materials or a similar chemical process.

Smoke detector: A device that automatically sounds an alarm when exposed to smoke.

Having a working smoke detector in your home can reduce your risk of death from a residential fire by 50 percent.

FIGURE 5.2
Locations of Smoke Detectors

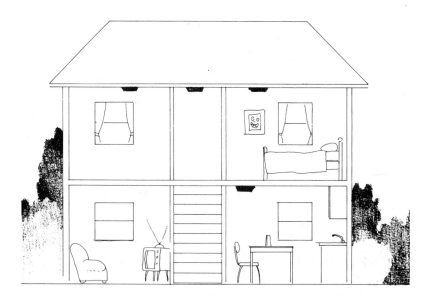

Smoke detectors should be installed in every level of a house and should be mounted high on the wall or on the ceiling, as smoke rises. Avoid locations near stoves, ovens, or close to a shower where steam or smoke is likely to produce a large number of false alarms. It is particularly important to place detectors near sleeping areas, as the risk of undetected fire is greatest at night.

bedrooms. The National Fire Protection Association recommends that detectors also be placed in other highly used areas, such as living rooms and hallways.

Detectors should be installed on the ceiling (at least 4 inches from the wall) or high on the wall (4 to 12 inches from the ceiling). Do not place detectors near a stove or oven or close to the shower; the steam from hot water or food can inadvertently set off the alarm. If the alarm is battery operated, change the batteries every year on a date you will remember, such as your birthday or when daylight-saving time ends. Be sure to read the instruction manual included with your unit.

EMERGENCY PLAN

When fire occurs, knowing how to exit the house safely becomes crucial. The National Fire Prevention Association recommends that every family develop an emergency plan that contains the following points:

1. Draw a floor plan of your home and indicate all exit routes.

2. Teach all family members to check doors before opening them. If a doorknob is hot, use an alternate route. If it is cool, open the door slowly and carefully.

3. If smoke is entering a room under a door, stuff rags or towels under the door and in the cracks.

4. Know in advance who will take small children and infants out of the house.

5. Stay low in an effort to keep from breathing smoke and hot air. If possible, crawl on hands and knees.

(continued on p. 103)

Save Your Family From a Fire

It's the middle of the night. You're sound asleep—until the piercing sound of the smoke alarm jolts you awake. Now what do you do? Try to find the fire? Get dressed? Grab all the valuables? The answer is, before you do anything, wake everyone up.

If you are like most Americans, you may be ill-prepared to handle an emergency fire situation effectively. However, you need not be defenseless in the face of a fire in your home. The amount of attention that you pay to fire safety can be the key to your family's survival.

"People can cut their risk of dying in a fire in half by using smoke detectors," notes Jamie Haines, spokesperson for the National Fire Protection Association (NFPA).

Fireproofing your home.

According to the International Association of Fire Chiefs, although three out of four American households have at least one smoke detector, as many as half of those in place are not working. Some have dead batteries or no batteries at all. The peak months for home fires are December and January, the holiday season. Often batteries are "borrowed" from smoke detectors for Christmas toys or other appliances and are never replaced. Batteries should be checked at least every month and changed at least once a year. Intermittent chirping sounds may mean that batteries are fading. (It may be easier to remember to change batteries if you do it on your birthday or when you change your clocks for daylight saving time.)

Contrary to popular belief, victims of fire often never even smell smoke. Before they're aware that there's smoke in the house, most are asphyxiated by the smoke and toxic gases that numb the senses and induce a deeper sleep. Therefore, the rousing sound of a smoke alarm is especially critical at night, when most home fires occur.

Notes Jamie Haines of the NFPA, "People are

lulled into a false sense of security by thinking that if they have a smoke detector in their home, even a nonfunctioning one, they are somehow protected against fire." Likewise, parents often have a distorted sense of their own innate abilities to handle emergency situations involving their children; most have the notion that they will leap into action at the first sign of smoke to save their kids. But, often, it's the smoke that prevents you from getting to a child's room.

For your safety and your children's safety, the NFPA recommends that you and your children sleep with your bedroom doors closed. While young children often don't like this sleeping arrangement, it is crucial that parents realize that a child's closed door may be the key factor in saving his life in a fire. A closed door can keep the deadly smoke and fire at bay for valuable minutes until help arrives.

It is also imperative that you have smoke alarms on every level of your home, including the basement, according to the U.S. Fire Administration. At the very least you should have smoke detectors outside and inside each bedroom. For the most protection, the NFPA recommends also putting detectors in the dining room, furnace room, and hallways.

Because smoke rises, filling the highest points of the house before making its way to the floor, it is necessary to mount smoke alarms high on walls or on ceilings. Detectors should be installed on the ceiling at least four inches from each wall or on a wall four to twelve inches from the ceiling. Avoid placing alarms near windows, air vents, fans, or air conditioners, where drafts can prevent smoke from entering the detector. Similarly, do not place a detector above the stove or near the shower, because it will be set off constantly. Resist the urge to disarm a smoke alarm that is triggered falsely. Fanning the steam or smoke away from the device or opening a nearby window is a far safer alternative than removing the batteries.

Smoke detectors must also be cleaned periodically, preferably once a year. Use the hose attachment of your vacuum cleaner to clean your detectors.

In addition to installing smoke detectors, you should consider having a residential sprinkling system put into your home. Sprinkler devices can be installed for about 90 cents to $3.50 per square foot, depending on the age of your home. The sprinkler system sprays water automatically in the area of the fire, before it can spread.

You also might consider investing in a couple of home fire extinguishers for key areas in the home, such as the kitchen or the workshop. However, Thomas Siegfried, fire chief of the Altamonte Springs Fire Department, in Florida, adds, "a $20 fire extinguisher can be helpful, but it is better to become adept at getting out of the house."

An escape plan.

Make a step-by-step, room-to-room survey of your home. First, make sure there are two ways out of every room. One exit will be the regular entrance or door to the hallway, for instance, while the second will probably be a window. (The second way out is needed in case smoke and fire fill the hallway and block the primary exit.) Decide who will get young children out of the house, and establish a meeting place *outside* the home, preferably at a landmark such as a tree or mailbox, where the family can gather to regroup.

Double-check the exits you have designated, and conduct a walk-through of your house. Examine windows and doors. Do all windows open easily? Are there warped doors that won't close completely? Are you familiar with how to open storm windows? Can you reach the ground from a window exit? If not, you should have an Underwriters Laboratories, Inc., "UL Listed" safety ladder or a rope ladder at each window that is not accessible to a balcony, deck, or garage roof.

Make sure to plan how *every* family member can reach the ground from an emergency exit. Decide which parent will be responsible for finding an infant or toddler and which parent will go out the bedroom window or door to get help. You don't want both of you running to retrieve the same child in a panic.

If you live in an apartment, you also need to be familiar with two ways out of the apartment as well as the route to the enclosed exit stairs.

Practice unlocking a deadbolt quickly. Do not use locks that require keys to open the door from the inside. Don't ever get into an elevator to escape a fire, because it may take you right to the fire, or the power may fail and you can become trapped inside the elevator. Use the stairwell. Shut all doors behind you; do not leave them propped open for the people behind you. Smoke and fumes can fill a stairwell in three minutes, possibly killing you and those behind you as well. If you have a fire escape covered by a gate in your apartment, make sure the gate is fire department–approved and can be easily opened from the outside.

Fire drills.

Family fire drills should be held regularly, and baby-sitters should be involved occasionally in the exercise. "You don't want the first time you wonder how to escape to be when that smoke alarm goes off for real," says Gordon Routley, assistant to the fire chief of Phoenix, Arizona. You have only minutes to evacuate your family once the alarm sounds. A smoke detector does not go off until the smoke has reached a certain level. Therefore, smoke has already been accumulating for some time by the time the alarm sounds.

Children under five are most at risk of dying in a house fire, so it is critical to equip preschoolers with the tools that will help them survive. For example, children need to learn what to expect when the smoke alarm sounds. Otherwise, they could panic and instinctively try to run and hide in an enclosed space, such as under a bed or in a closet, where they erroneously believe they will be safe. Or a child may hide because he thinks that he has done something wrong and that he himself is responsible for the alarm. Tragically, most children who die in fires are found lying under beds or in closets.

Children need to be taught a home escape plan in the event of a fire. Depending on the child's physical and mental maturity, she should be told either to wait by the window to be rescued or to go out the primary or secondary exit on her own.

"In order for the fire drill to be effective, it is important that family members actually go out that window and down that ladder when rehearsing," emphasizes Jamie Haines of the NFPA. Find out if your child needs a footstool to reach her window and if she feels comfortable opening her window by herself. "It makes a tremendous difference if families have practiced trying to get out," says Haines. "If kids don't know they can do this, the chances that they'll panic are greater."

You can teach fire safety skills to children the way you teach them about seat belts. Use hard facts, not scare tactics. It is important that a child knows there are specific steps she can take to empower herself if fire strikes.

How fires start.

It is important to stress to children the danger of playing with matches and cigarette lighters. When a child is five, try sitting him down and teaching him how to light a match, suggests Leora Bowden, senior social worker at the University of Michigan Burn Center, in Ann Arbor. Explain to your child that a match is not a toy but a tool that is to be used only when an adult is present. Tell him that anytime he gets the urge to light a match he can come to you and do it in front of you. "Because matches are everywhere and kids have a tendency to be curious and intrigued by fire, you are lessening the attraction to the forbidden element of playing with matches," adds Bowden. Let your child know how proud you are that he is fire safety-conscious. Of course, you still should never leave matches and cigarette lighters where kids can reach them.

There are numerous ways in which fires can start besides kids' playing with matches. Many home fires begin in the kitchen, where you and your family should be especially vigilant and safety-conscious. The NFPA offers the following lifesaving household tips.

In the kitchen. Wear tight shirtsleeves when you cook, since loose sleeves can catch fire easily. Don't store items on or over the stove, because you can get burned reaching across the stove. Be wary of deep-frying or cooking with grease. Heat oil slowly, never on high. Do not use water to put out a grease fire. Put out the fire by placing the pan lid over the pan and turning off the burner or by dousing the flame with lots of baking soda. If a fire starts in the oven, shut the oven door to put out the fire, and then turn off the heat. Don't leave pot holders on the stove, and never leave your house when you have something cooking on the stove. Finally, keep your stove and oven clean, because accumulated grease and food particles can catch fire readily. For a fire that starts in your microwave oven, quickly shut the door and press the Stop button. If you open the door, you will only fan the fire.

Also, remember not to overload your electrical sockets by plugging in too many appliances at once. Replace any cords that are frayed or cracked. Turn off appliances after using them, as coffeepots and toaster ovens, for instance, can overheat and start a fire.

Heating equipment. According to the NFPA, accidents with heating equipment are the number one cause of fires in the home, so make sure portable heaters are placed at least three feet away from anything that can burn. They should also have a child-proof guard around them. Always turn off portable heaters when you leave home and before going to bed. Use only wood in a fireplace or wood-burning stove. Remember that heaters should be used only when adults are present.

Family rooms. In the living room and family room offer ashtrays to smokers, and always check under sofa and chair cushions for smoldering cigarettes before going to bed. (A cigarette butt can smolder for five hours before bursting into flames while you sleep.) Fill ashtrays with water before disposing of cigarette butts, and never smoke in bed! Have chimneys cleaned regularly, and always use a screen on the hearth. Allow at least one foot of space between the wall and electronic equipment as well as between each piece of furniture.

In the basement. In the basement or garage make sure gasoline and other flammable liquids

are not stored near a heat source. Don't store anything near a furnace or heater, and have your furnace checked every year.

Don't substitute a penny for or wrap foil around an old blown fuse, as this can lead to overheating and fire. Keep a supply of appropriate size fuses on hand.

Proceed with caution.
Despite your taking these safety steps, fires can still break out. If a fire does start in your home, remember that countless lives have been lost because people have gone back inside a burning house and died from one deep breath of toxic fumes and smoke. "You don't want to jeopardize your own safety so that you are unable to get the help needed to save your family," stresses Jamie Haines. Firefighters have the necessary clothing, equipment, and training to go into a burning house. Your job is to get out and call the fire department. You are better off if you can teach every member of your family his own role in the fire escape plan and then make sure that each person sticks to it.

Firefighters will search every room to find someone who is still in a house, notes Routley. "Tot Finder" stickers can alert firefighters to where children are located and may help to guide them in their search.

However, Routley says, "stickers promote complacency and a false sense of security." Teaching a young child to wait at the window of his room to be rescued is the best way to help the firefighters find him.

Fires are something you hate to think about, but they do happen. You'll sleep a little easier knowing you have done everything in your power to make your home and family fire-safe.

Jan Hart Sousa is a Connecticut-based freelance writer and the mother of 3 children, ages 8, 5, and 3 months.

Source: *Parents*, October 1989, pp. 82–89.

6. Establish a meeting place outside the home, such as a tree, mailbox, or other landmark, so the family can gather after exiting the house.

7. Once everyone has exited safely, no one should return to rescue pets or valuables.

Hold fire drills periodically so all members of the family know what to do in specific cases. Check to see that all escape routes are accessible and that all exits (such as windows) can be opened. During the drills, it is important that all members of the family actually go out the exits, especially if they must go out a window or climb down a ladder. Do not wait until a fire occurs to see if the procedure works.

EXTINGUISHING FIRES

Fires are classified into 4 categories according to composition and severity:

Class A fires are fueled by ordinary combustible materials such as wood, paper, rubbish, cloth, and some plastics. The most commonly used extinguishing agent for this type of fire is water, which cools the fuel.

Class B fires are fueled by flammable liquids such as grease, oil, gasoline, kerosene, and alcohol. This type of fire should be smothered or should be doused with a combustion-inhibiting agent such as a dry chemical, foam, or carbon dioxide.

Class C fires are fires involving energized electrical equipment or wires. Extinguishing agents must be nonconductors such as a dry chemical, carbon dioxide, or **halogenated hydrocarbons (Halon)**. Water, foam, and water-type agents are good conductors of electricity; their use can injure or kill the person operating the extinguisher.

Class D fires involve combustible metals such as magnesium, titanium, zirconium, and sodium. These metals are usually found in industrial settings and require special techniques and equipment to extinguish. Normal extinguishing agents should not be used because they may actually increase the intensity of the fire.

Naturally, the most important thing to do *immediately* after a fire has been detected is to get yourself and your family out of the house and away from the flame. Next call for help. Do not try to extinguish the flame yourself unless you are confident of your ability to do so. Cooling a fire requires the application of an agent

Halogenated hydrocarbons (Halon): Organically based chemicals formed by combining one or more hydrocarbons with one or more of the halogen elements—fluorine, chlorine, iodine, bromine, or astatine; such compounds are highly effective extinguishing agents, particularly for electrical (class C) fires.

that absorbs heat. Water is the most common of these agents. Application is usually by a hose stream, fog, fine spray, or foam. The 3 basic methods of extinguishing a fire are as follows:

1. *Removal of Fuel:* Sometimes the best way to extinguish a fire is to remove the fuel. This may entail turning off the gas

The Fundamentals of Fire Extinguishment

FIRE	Fire burns because three elements are present—heat, fuel and oxygen. In technical language, fire is a chemical reaction: It happens when a material unites with oxygen so rapidly that it produces flame. Think of fire as a triangle. If any one of three sides—heat, fuel or oxygen—is taken away, the fire goes out. This is the basis for fire extinguishment. Heat can be taken away by cooling, oxygen can be taken away by excluding air, fuel can be removed to a place where there is no flame, chemical reaction can be stopped by inhibiting the oxidation of the fuel.
REMOVE HEAT	Cooling a fire calls for the application of something which absorbs heat. Although there are others, water is the most common cooling agent. Water is commonly applied in the form of a solid stream, finely divided spray or incorporated in foam.
REMOVE FUEL	Often, taking the fuel away from a fire is difficult and dangerous, but there are exceptions. Flammable liquid storage tanks can be arranged so their contents can be pumped to an isolated empty tank in case of fire. When flammable gases catch fire as they are flowing from a pipe, the fire will go out if the flow can be valved off.
REMOVE OXYGEN	Oxygen can be taken away from a fire by covering it with a wet blanket, throwing dirt on it or covering it with chemical or mechanical foam. Other gases which are heavier than air, such as carbon dioxide and vaporizing liquid, can be used to blanket the fire, preventing the oxygen from getting to the fire.
STOP THE REACTION	Studies made during recent years have indicated that the familiar statement, "Remove heat, remove fuel, or remove oxygen, to extinguish a fire" does not apply when dry chemical or halogenated hydrocarbons are used as the extinguishing agents. These agents inactivate intermediate products of the flame reaction resulting in a reduction of the combustion rate, [which] extinguishes the fire.

Source: The Ansul Company, Marinette, Wisconsin.

FIGURE 5.3
Use of a Fire Extinguisher

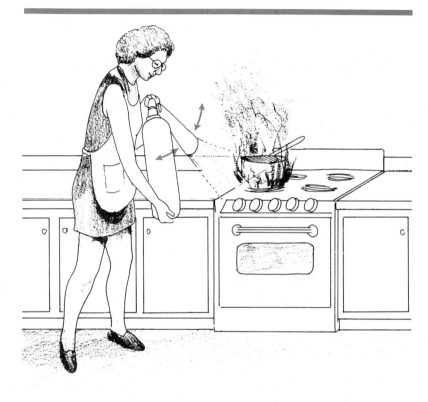

When using a fire extinguisher, always aim it at the base of the flames and use a sweeping motion to cover the entire area that is burning.

flowing through a gas pipe or using a bulldozer to create a firebreak across the path of an approaching forest fire.

2. *Removal of Oxygen:* Smothering a fire by putting a lid on a burning skillet, throwing a wet blanket over a fire, or throwing dirt or sand on the flame are all ways of removing oxygen from a fire. Gases that are heavier than air, such as carbon dioxide, can blanket the fire and keep the oxygen out.

3. *Interruption of the Chain Reaction:* Using a dry chemical or Halon on a fire interrupts the chain reaction and extinguishes the flame.

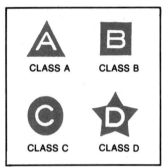

CLASS A   CLASS B

CLASS C   CLASS D

Portable Fire Extinguishers

Most home **fire extinguishers** are designed to put out the 3 types of fires that can occur in the home: Classes A, B, and C (common combustible, flammable liquids, and electrical). However, not all extinguishers are effective for all 3, so it is important to read the label. Some labels use a letter system— A, B, C, or D. Others use letters and symbols—the symbol for Class A is a green triangle; for Class B, a red square; for Class C, a blue circle; and for Class D, a yellow star. [4]

Operating an Extinguisher

Although portable fire extinguishers vary in size and shape, they all operate in much the same way. The first thing to do when using an extinguisher is to break the seal and pull the pin. Do this immediately, before you get to the fire, if possible. Stay low and hold the extinguisher in an upright position. Aim the stream at the base of the flame and use a sweeping motion to cover the entire fire. Be careful not to waste any of the agent; many extinguishers have only 15 to 60 seconds of discharge. Finally, remember that portable fire extinguishers have their limitations. Do not try to fight large fires with them. Instead, call the fire department immediately.

(continued on p. 109)

Fire extinguisher: A device designed to put out small-to-moderate-sized fires quickly.

Yes, Virginia, There Is a Fire Problem

Fire in the United States, the subject of the comprehensive [seventh] edition of the U.S. Fire Administration's yearly report, provides some hope for reducing the nation's fire losses, but highlights the fact that much remains to be done. The reason for hope is a slight downward trend in the number of fires, the number of deaths, and even (after taking into account the effects of inflation) the dollar value of property lost by fire. However, even with the recent improvements, this country continues to maintain the third highest per capita loss by fire among all nations in the industrialized world. This publication highlights figures of that loss—based on data from 1983[–1988], and published in July [1990], by the U.S. Fire Administration.

There were an estimated 2.[1] million fires in the United States in [1989]. Those fires claimed some 6,100 lives and injured 110,000 people. An estimated [$10.4] billion was lost. This placed the United States (in deaths per million population) third among the industrialized nations of the world behind Scotland and Canada. These figures equate to 2.5 deaths and 45 injuries per 1,000 fires. The average property loss per fire was [$4,700].

Our nation's fire losses in 1983 were better than average for recent years. In fact, the figures have been gradually diminishing since 1977, when the United States suffered an estimated 16.2 fires per 1,000 population. The figure for 1983 was 9.9 fires per 1,000 population. Losses of life and property have gradually diminished, as well. For example, an estimated 39.2 Americans lost their lives for each one million people in 1974. That figure . . . gradually declined to 27 deaths per million Americans in 1983.

As in the past, the greatest burden among fire

causalities was borne by the very young and the very old—ages zero to 4 and 65 and older. Men are about twice as likely to die in a fire as are women; blacks and Native Americans have extremely high death rates. Chinese, Japanese, and other Asians have inordinately low death rates. Firefighters face a substantial risk of death and injury in fighting fires.

Residential fires form the core of the fire problem in the United States. They cause three-fourths of the nation's fire-related deaths and two-thirds of the fire-related injuries. Almost half of all property losses occur in residential fires.

Most (79 percent) residential fires occur in one- or two-family homes. Apartments, flats and tenements account for 18 percent.

The important lesson for everyone concerned with fires in this type of facility is that much can be done for a relatively small cost. Smoke detectors should be mandatory. Walls and ceilings can be protected with an interior finish of limited combustibility—especially in hallways, entrances and exits. The effectiveness of such measures can be dramatic: In a fire in a group home in Eau Claire, Wis., there were two exits—one was protected and the other was not. Residents who used the unprotected exit died or sustained severe injuries; those who used the protected exit escaped unharmed.

A relatively inexpensive sprinkler system in hallways and exits can keep passageways tenable while residents are escaping. Here is an example from *Fire in the United States:*

Following two severe residential fires in Washington, D.C., the U.S. Fire Administration offered a special grant program so that sprinkler systems could be placed in several similar facilities. Recently, a fire broke out in one of the houses so protected. The scenario of this fire was similar to that of the other two fires, which had resulted in a total of 15 fatalities, in that it occurred late at night and was caused by an ignition factor where smoking materials ignited textiles.

The third incident had a significant difference, however, as the sprinkler system went into operation and extinguished the fire. There were no deaths, no serious injuries, and damage was confined to a couch and the area immediately surrounding it. Water damage from the sprinkler system was minimal and, needless to say, far less than had a fire department been called to extinguish the blaze.

Fires in most categories of institutional buildings have been a relatively minor problem. The incidence of school fires, for example, has greatly diminished in recent years because of safer construction methods and materials, and safer school practices. Although there were 6,600 reported school fires in 1983, there was only one death.

One of the most hopeful notes in America's fire loss experience in recent years has been the steady decline in the number of firefighters who have lost their lives. America lost 170 firefighters in 1978; that figure has steadily declined to [105] in [1990]. Of those [105], nearly half lost their lives while fighting fires. Slightly less than a quarter died while they were responding to calls; the remainder were killed in the course of training or while performing other types of emergency or routine duties. . . .

"Better training, improved equipment, and a heightened awareness for issues of health and safety have helped reduce this tragic toll," said Edward Wall, deputy administrator of the U.S. Fire Administration.

A less hopeful trend in recent years has been that of fire incidents caused by alternative sources of home heating. Over the past 10 years, alternative methods of heating homes have increased dramatically. The increased use of both portable- and fixed-heating devices has seen a concomitant rise in the number of fires associated with these devices. This has been especially true in homes where the alternative heating system was the *only* heating system in use.

Probably the most vexing problem faced by the nation's firefighting community is arson. The exact number of cases of arson each year is not known. However, both the Federal Bureau of Investigation's Uniform Crime Reporting System and the National Fire Protection Association report that arson rates have been virtually unchanged in recent years. On a national scale, according to U.S. Fire Administration projections, arson accounts for about 400,000 fires, 850 deaths, 23,000 injuries, and $1.4 billion in damages annually.

The last decade has brought progress in the area of eliminating clothing fires. Prior to the mid-60s, clothing fires were an especially dangerous threat to children and seniors. Research concluding that flammable fabrics played a major role in this type of fire has resulted in regulations governing flammability standards in clothing and children's sleepwear.

The U.S. Fire Administration attempts to identify, from the information it gathers each year, those areas that warrant special consideration. Here are the salient areas that should be watched:

• *Boarding and rooming houses*—These houses are often inadequately maintained from the standpoint of fire prevention and safety. The risk of death from these fires is 27 per 1,000 fires, as compared with 7.2 per 1,000 fires in other residential categories.

• *Alternative heaters*—Solid fuel heating equipment is the largest single source of fires in one- and two-family homes. Although portable space heaters cause relatively few fires, the risk of death in a space heater fire is about 10 times the national average (for all fires) and about six times the average for a residential fire. . . .

• *Envelope houses*—These are constructed for energy efficiency, and are positioned partially underground. Preliminary evidence suggests that these super-insulated homes suffer from fires that are inordinately intense—possibly because they allow less heat to escape.

• *Cabinet heaters*—This is an area that bears special attention in the immediate future. These heaters, long available in Europe, house a 20-pound rechargeable propane cylinder. The domestic gas industry has expressed a strong interest in marketing the heaters in the United States.

The foremost concern is the risk when they are overfilled. If a unit is filled in a cold outdoor storage area, and then brought into a warm area, the resulting excess pressure in the heater could trigger the relief valve that would then release LP gas into the user's home. The relief valve could also be triggered if the unit were heated by a fire on a lower floor. If the escaping gas reached an ongoing fire, it would, of course, ignite. Fire analysts are also concerned about the possibilities of faulty connections and users connecting the heaters to 40-pound LP cartridges, commonly used for gas barbecues.

Fire departments throughout the country have developed hundreds—even thousands—of imaginative, effective ways to communicate fire-safety lessons and awareness to their communities. Children in kindergartens have learned about the sounds that their "friends," the smoke detectors, make. In Louisville, Ky., children in more than 360 public schools have taken part in an event in which they have the opportunity to compete for a prize. Their fire-safety messages are written on stamped, self-addressed postcards and attached to helium-filled balloons. The balloons are released at the "Great Louisville Fire Drill," held at a local park. Anyone finding the balloons is requested (in a note on the postcard) to mail the postcard. The winning child is the one whose postcard is returned from the greatest distance.

Such programs, designed to meet the needs of each locality, are an effective means of reducing the number of deaths and injuries from fire. But practically any community could benefit from what is perhaps the simplest and least expensive fire prevention measure of all—the smoke detector. The greatest loss from both deaths and injuries arises from fires in the home. When a fire claims the life of someone who does not have a working smoke detector, the loss is a special kind of tragedy. It is inexcusable. To be sure, the smoke detector cannot totally prevent the loss of life or property. It cannot prevent all injuries due to fire. But the absence of a smoke detector is an error that is so great in its relationship to human life and suffering, that this area is an appropriate focus for all who are concerned with helping to ease the burden of fire in America. Working smoke detectors in every home is a goal that is attainable. America can well afford the cost. It absolutely cannot afford the alternative.

FEMA

Source: Federal Emergency Management Agency.

OCCUPATIONAL SAFETY

Many accidents that happen in the workplace are similar to those that occur elsewhere; falls and poisonings can happen on the job as well as in the home, and professional drivers can and do suffer motor vehicle accidents while working. Together, these resulted in 10,400 deaths in 1989 (see figure 5.4). Having examined these topics in previous chapters, we will not address them further here. Another safety concern in the workplace, however, does merit attention. This is **occupational illness**, which can result from certain health hazards encountered on the job.

Health Hazards

Millions of people in all types of industries are routinely exposed to conditions that can lead to illness.

Occupational diseases have 5 common causes: (1) contact with **carcinogens**, corrosives, bacteria, and solvents that can produce skin diseases; (2) contact with air pollutants such as dust, gases, vapors, and mists; (3) physical stresses such as noise, temperature, vibration, radiation, and lasers; (4) contact with biological agents such as molds and fungi; and (5) **ergonomic** stresses that include repetitive motion and poor worker-machine interaction.

Among the more significant occupational illnesses are the following:

Asbestosis: This disease is caused by exposure to **asbestos**. Asbestos is now known to cause cancer of the lungs, the chest and abdominal cavities, the stomach, and the intestines. Most victims of asbestos-induced cancers were exposed to asbestos over a long period of time. However, there is now strong evidence that even one day's exposure to large amounts of asbestos can damage the lungs. Results of studies involving asbestosis have prompted a national, top-priority effort to remove asbestos from workplaces, public buildings, and schools.

If you have reason to believe there is asbestos in your place of business, your home, or any other structure, contact a professional for evaluation. Evaluating and removing asbestos requires certified professionals. It is not a do-it-yourself project.

Other Cancers: Carcinogens in the workplace, such as coal tar products, a variety of toxic heavy metals, dyes, and a long list of other chemicals, can also cause cancer. Again, the presence of any of these substances calls for a professional search and evaluation.

Contact Dermatitis: **Contact dermatitis** is caused by skin exposure to resins, solvents, acids, oils, biological agents, dust,

Occupational illness: Any illness caused by conditions or hazards found in the workplace.

Carcinogen: Any substance known to cause cancer.

Ergonomic: Pertaining to the interaction of people and things.

Asbestos: A naturally occurring fibrous mineral widely used for insulation and fireproofing; prolonged exposure to asbestos has been linked to lung cancer and other diseases of the lung.

Contact dermatitis: A skin irritation resulting from exposure to nickel, detergents, medications, and a variety of other chemicals or substances.

FIGURE 5.4
Work-Related Deaths and Death Rates

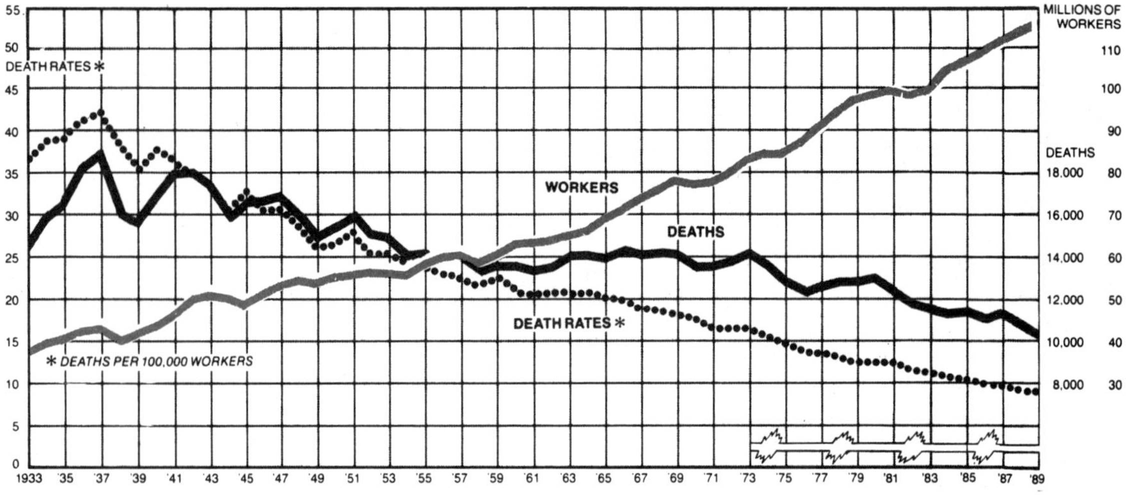

Source: National Safety Council, *Accident Facts*, 1990, p. 34.

As the above figure indicates, both the total number of accidental work deaths and the accidental work death rate have declined steadily in the United States throughout most of this century. Even so, work-related accidents resulted in some 10,400 deaths during 1989.

Silicosis: A lung disease caused by the inhalation of silica dust; it is characterized by shortness of breath and decreased chest expansion and is most common among workers over 50; acute cases may develop after as little as 10 months of continuous exposure.

Carpal tunnel syndrome: A condition characterized by numbness, tingling, or pain in the hands resulting from nerve damage caused by the swelling of inflamed tendons and membranes in the wrist; it is associated with jobs that require repetitive motion.

and other materials. The symptoms of dermatitis include a reddening of the skin, skin irritation, and a skin rash with mild or intense itching. Severe cases produce open sores as well as other complications.

Hearing Loss: Chronic exposure to noise and/or vibration can damage the hearing. Noise causes a substantial number of occupational illnesses. All susceptible employees should wear ear-protection equipment during working hours.

Silicosis: **Silicosis** is caused by breathing air containing silica dust, which causes thickening and scarring of the lungs. This in turn leads to shortness of breath, decreased chest expansion, and decreased ability to work. Silicosis is a problem primarily for workers in occupations such as quartz mining and blasting, and in the glass, ceramic, and stonecutting industries.

Carpal Tunnel Syndrome: **Carpal tunnel syndrome** occurs when inflamed tendons and membranes in the wrist swell and damage nerves that control finger and hand movement. Repeti-

FIGURE 5.5
Health Hazards in the Office

Did You Know That . . .

U.S. employees are more likely to die from workplace accidents than people in other industrialized countries—5 times more likely than Swedes, and 3 times more than Japanese.

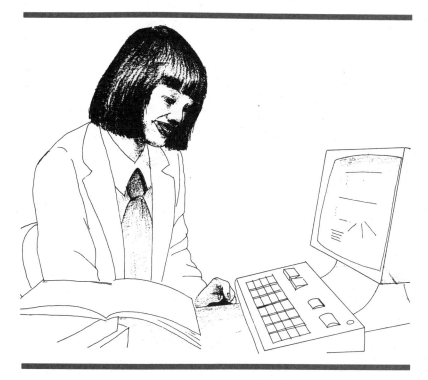

Even office work carries the risk of occupational illness. Some studies suggest that the electromagnetic fields emitted by video display terminals may cause health problems. It is recommended that users keep their monitors at arm's length and that they position themselves several feet away from other monitors in the office.

tive motion jobs, such as component assembly, meat cutting, computer keyboarding, and sorting operations, can all cause this condition.

Raynaud's Phenomenon: The primary symptom of **Raynaud's phenomenon** is a numbness and blanching of the fingers. Although it has several possible causes, it is a recognized occupational disorder of workers who use pneumatic, electrical, or gasoline power tools whose operation exposes them to prolonged vibration. It is a progressive disease and in most cases irreversible.

Controlling Hazardous Environmental Problems
Responsible employers make a serious attempt to reduce their

Raynaud's phenomenon: A blood vessel disorder characterized by the sudden contraction of the small arteries in the fingers and toes on exposure to cold resulting in their turning white, often accompanied by a feeling of numbness or tingling.

(continued on p. 115)

Danger on the Job

José Americano Guzman helped get 18-year-old Juan Carlos Roque his job at the Star Scrap Metal Co. in La Mirada, Calif. They were cousins, but their 13-year age difference made it feel more like a protective uncle-nephew relationship. A few weeks after starting work, Roque was cleaning out a metal-compacting machine, a task some companies make safe by "locking out" the on/off switch during maintenance. This company didn't, and Roque was sliced in half when the machine was accidentally turned on—by his cousin José.

Roughly 120 people die each year from similar "lock out" accidents, just one of many types of ghoulish and preventable job-related deaths. Workplace death, illness and injury don't get nearly the attention of dramatic disasters, but the human costs are, in fact, much greater. Take the death toll for the five worst floods in America since 1925, add the fatalities from the five worst hurricanes, the five worst tornadoes, then the earthquakes, plane crashes, train wrecks and fires. All those casualities number far fewer than the 21,000 workers who died from workplace accidents in 1987 and 1988, according to the National Safety Council. And that's just from accidents. Estimates are that many more die from illnesses caused by workplace hazards.

Work is safer than it was 50 years ago. And most workplace accidents do not involve deaths. But occupational safety and health experts say large sectors of the economy have hardly improved in the last 20 years, and some have gotten worse. Reminders of the work risks come regularly. [In a recent] week four construction workers and a bus driver died when a crane toppled from the 16th floor of a San Francisco high-rise. October [1989's] Phillips Petroleum explosion in Pasadena, Texas, which killed 23 workers and injured more than 100, was only the most dramatic in a recent rash of oil-refining and petrochemical disasters.

Workers, according to a recent survey by a management-consulting firm, list safety as their No. 1 job priority, ahead of salary, benefits or day care. Under the direction of Labor Secretary Elizabeth Dole, the Occupational Safety and Health Administration (OSHA) has shown new energy. The effort couldn't come at a better time. [In November 1989] the Bureau of Labor Statistics announced that the reported injury rate rose in 1988, continuing a trend that began in 1983. Officials say some of the increases result from more accurate reporting by companies that fear OSHA sanctions. But that doesn't mitigate the problem: injuries are either more numerous, or are worse than we thought.

The most hazardous industry in America is not petrochemicals, construction, mining or manufacturing. It is farming. In 1988, 1,500 agricultural workers died—nearly twice the rate of miners—and there were 140,000 disabling injuries. Agriculture also has the highest rate of poisonings, skin diseases and respiratory conditions due to toxic agents, according to the National Safety Council. Too little awareness of hazards and the absence of regulation explain some of the bad record. Wary of federal involvement in farm safety, agriculture groups have had OSHA banned from regulating or even recording deaths for more than 95 percent of farms. Says Jack King of the American Farm Bureau Federation, "The last thing [farmers] want to do is get encumbered in a lot of paperwork."

Some farmers remove safety shields from machinery for convenience or just don't realize that ordinary functions pose lethal dangers. In 1980 Randy Claussen of Bettendorf, Iowa, went into a partially enclosed manure pit to unclog a pump and was overcome by poisonous hydrogen sulfide fumes. Claussen's father went in to save his son but collapsed as well. Another son followed, and when firefighters arrived they found all three dead. Greater awareness of accidents might prevent them, but it's unlikely that farmers would hear the details of tragedies two states away. The federal government now spends only 30 cents per farmer on safety education annually, compared with $4.48 for industry and $244 for mining.

Most disturbingly, children make up more than a fifth of agricultural fatalities. More than half are killed when they fall off or are run over by tractors. A recent survey offered an ironic explanation: parents put kids on machinery to get them interested in agriculture. "Can you imagine if USX or Exxon were to report that last year there were 40 kids killed in their refineries?" asks Bill Field, an agriculture safety expert at Purdue University.

In some cases, workplace injuries have increased because of seemingly healthy economic or social forces. John Morrell & Co. has increased productivity in its Sioux Falls, S.D., meat-processing plant since 1979 by having workers perform simple, narrow tasks over and over. But "repetitive motion injuries," potentially crippling tendon and muscle afflictions, jumped dramatically at the same time. Technological innovation has also brought more of these injuries to the office. Clean, efficient computers have led to more wrist injuries than typewriters, whose clunkiness forced typists to make fuller use of their arms.

Risks to rookies: Injuries also tend to rise when the economy expands, as some companies hire less experienced workers without providing extra safety precautions. . . . Mickey Albritten had been on the job for just four days at Cagle's poultry-processing plant in Macon, Ga., and, at 5 foot 3, he was straining to hang chickens on an overhead conveyor line. He says he hadn't been given safety training, and when his thumb got caught in the belt no one else was around to hear his screams. The machine pulled him along the plant floor and was lifting him by his thumb into the air toward a partition. Albritten panicked and pulled off his own finger. Cagle's issued a statement noting that it has since installed an on/off switch near the belt and that "any employee who requests hand wraps or over-the-counter [painkillers] is readily supplied with them."

Some patterns of workplace injury haven't changed for a century: recent immigrants are less likely to complain about work conditions. In Los Angeles County, 40 percent of workplace fatalities involve non-English speakers. Regulators fear that intense international competition and an influx of new immigrants have helped dramatically increase the number of textile sweatshops with chemical and fire hazards.

OSHA, the agency charged with solving these problems, has had a troubled history. Created in 1971, it was just starting to figure out how to regulate well when it fell victim to deregulation a decade later. Citing nit-picky rules, like one from the mid-1970s requiring toilet seats to be horseshoe shaped, the Reagan administration persuaded Congress to approve budgets that shrank OSHA's staff. The Office of Management and Budget stalled key regulations. In 1982, OSHA inspectors checked the books of the Film Recovery Systems, a company that extracted the silver out of old X-ray film, in Elk Grove Village, Ill., but because of a practice limiting on-scene inspections they didn't visit a nearby building, where cyanide was killing one worker and making others seriously ill. Even after it did announce the imposition of fines, OSHA would negotiate them down, on average to one third their original level, according to a National Safe Workplace Institute study.

Record find: The agency, several longtime critics say, has improved dramatically under its new administrator, Gerard Scannell, and Labor Secretary Dole. It recently hit USX Corp. with a $7.3 million fine, the largest ever, alleging hundreds of violations including 58 "willful" hazards it claimed the steel giant knew about but didn't fix. The company is appealing the fine. Dole has speeded up proposals to reduce machine accidents, asphyxiations, AIDS hazards for health-care workers and motor-vehicle fatalities (the biggest cause of job-related death). Perhaps most important, she got the agency a major budget increase.

But even a rejuvenated OSHA can get at only a fraction of the problems. Most workplace deaths are not reported to OSHA. Scarce resources and legal restrictions make it difficult to regulate the millions of small businesses, some of which have high injury rates. Unions, which often spark investigations, now represent only 19 percent of the work force. And while federal OSHA has imposed more than 100 fines of over $100,000, 21 states regulate safety locally and have given out only a handful of the large penalties.

Scannell and Dole have tried to convince business that safety improves productivity and lowers insurance costs. Truth is, safety pays off but not necessarily right away. Reducing chemical exposure may cost money now while the effects of hazards might not be felt until years later when workers develop diseases. "When it really comes down to the crunch on the floor, production gets the nod over safety," says Scannell, formerly safety chief at Johnson & Johnson.

Some companies argue that the dangers are inherent in their industries. "We do everything we can," says Monte Janssen of the Texas Chemical Council. "But the bottom line is, an accident can happen." Safety experts also believe that drug or alcohol abuse, family problems or depression can lead to injuries by clouding workers' judgment, slowing their reflexes or causing sudden physical seizures. Many companies have responded by instituting drug testing. Investigators are looking at whether such problems helped cause the San Francisco crane accident. Lonnie Boggess, who operated the crane, was an alleged alcoholic who told a divorce hearing in 1989 that "the mistakes I was making were coming close to causing catastrophic injury to fellow employees." He said the Erection Co. laid him off once because of his mental state. He was later rehired for the San Francisco job. The company could not be reached for comment.

Life or limb: The best proof that workers' problems aren't the main reason for health and safety problems is that companies within the same industries have vastly different records. The Bechtel Group construction company has had only five fatalities in the last 490 million hours of work. Swinerton & Wallberg Co., the general contractor at the San Francisco crane site, has had nine fatalities in the last 4 million hours. Workers do make mistakes that help cause accidents. But most safety experts believe that management, training and workplace design determine whether the worker pays for his error

with life or limb. "I used to cringe when I'd hear managers say, 'I knew that guy was going to cut his finger off'," says the National Safety Council's Gary Fisher, formerly a safety manager at Martin Marietta. "Well [if you knew], why didn't you do anything about it? You would have if he had screwed up production."

Government and business seem to hold double standards when it comes to workplace safety. Regulators restrict the levels of toxic lead in the air. But step inside a workplace and the permissible level jumps 33 times. The Food and Drug Administration won't allow a cosmetic on the market before testing it. Yet a National Academy of Sciences study found that 60 percent of all chemicals used in the workplace had never been studied. Martin Marietta has a vice president for environmental affairs and a vice president for "ethics," but none for safety. The maximum prison term under federal law for polluting a stream is more than for negligently allowing a workplace death. The Environmental Protection Agency's budget is more than 21 times that of OSHA. Says John Moran, former safety director at the National Institute for Occupational Safety and Health: "Injury, illnesses and death in the workplace [are] still socially acceptable."

Workers themselves can, in some cases, decide whether the risks are worth it. Scallopers in Owls Head, Maine, joke that since they're going to die eventually, they would rather do it at sea. It's a line that doesn't amuse Deborah Damon, who has lost her grandfather, brother, former boyfriend and husband in fishing accidents. Why don't workers walk away from dangerous jobs? Some don't know the hazards. A jury in 1987 concluded that doctors at Du Pont Co. deliberately withheld health-related information from workers exposed to asbestos in Deepwater, N.J. Other workers psychologically discount the prospect of being killed because they can't afford to give up their jobs.

Tough choice: David DeLuise was faced with a tough choice when supervisors at Bethlehem Steel in October 1988 instructed him to use an unusually high-powered pump to push hot water through a cleaning tank unable to withstand great pressure. On the one hand, he seemed to know there was a risk. "Do you believe this? These bastards want me to use this as a back-wash pump," DeLuise told a co-worker. But De-Luise was on work probation, having completed an alcoholism-treatment program, and may have feared that refusing the order would cost him his job, friends say. So he turned on the pump. The tank exploded, doused him with scalding water and toxic chemicals, and seriously burned 95 percent of his body. His wife, Roxanne, says that "the only piece of the pillow you could see was an inch on either side of his head, he was that swollen. He would lie there, look at me and tears would roll out of his eyes." He survived for six weeks before dying.

Supervisors told other workers that drinking by DeLuise caused the accident, even though hospital blood tests found no trace of alcohol. "They treat their own employees and families like they don't even exist," Roxanne DeLuise says. Bethlehem spokesman Gary Graham refused to comment on the accident's cause, he said, to avoid "adding to [the family's] grief." But he said that the plant, which has had 20 deaths since 1972, now has a full-time safety director. OSHA, meanwhile, cited the company with a "serious" violation for allowing hazards "that were causing or likely to cause death or serious physical harm." They fined Bethlehem, a $4.6 billion company, $1,000, the legal maximum for that type of problem. DeLuise wants the health and safety laws changed because, she says, "an employer owes their employees a safe work environment." Fixing the laws will help, but little will really change until society starts placing a higher value on lives ruined or lost on the job.

Source: Steven Waldman et al., *Newsweek* (11 December 1989), pp. 42–46.

employees' exposure to environmental health hazards. These steps include:

1. Identifying potentially toxic materials and substituting less hazardous ones whenever possible

2. Designing the company's basic work processes to minimize employee exposure to hazardous situations

3. Isolating or otherwise limiting the number of employees exposed to an unavoidably dangerous process

4. Wetting dusty materials or using other methods to reduce dust

5. Providing adequate ventilation systems

6. Providing and encouraging the use of personal protective equipment, such as dust masks and goggles

7. Educating employees about specific occupational hazards

8. Setting up alarm and monitoring systems

9. Maintaining good housekeeping and storage, and disposing of all hazardous materials properly.

Safety Legislation for the Workplace

The campaign to prevent accidents in the workplace received a big boost in 1970 when the Williams-Steiger Occupational Safety and Health Act was enacted. Many people believe that this act was the most comprehensive legislation ever developed for worker safety. The law provides for establishment and enforcement of occupational safety and health standards covering workers across the nation. Under the Act the **Occupational Safety and Health Administration (OSHA)** was created within the U.S. Department of Labor. The law required businesses to establish a record-keeping system to monitor job-related injuries and illnesses, and authorized the new agency to develop safety and health standards for the protection of workers. It also established training and employee education programs and provided for mandatory inspections and strict penalties for companies which failed to comply with the newly established safety standards. In addition, the law established the **National Institute for Occupational Safety and Health (NIOSH)** in the Department of Health and Human Services for the purpose of conducting research and education programs.

Since its passage, the Act has elicited both praise and criticism. Many critics suggest that infrequent inspections and lack of general compliance serve as reasons to question the value of OSHA's performance. But studies in California and Wisconsin suggest that approximately 25 percent of work-related injuries could have been prevented had the businesses involved complied with OSHA standards. No doubt every workplace should do what it can to ensure safety for its employees. Following OSHA regulations is a good place to begin. W

Occupational Safety and Health Administration (OSHA): An office of the U.S. Department of Labor that monitors job-related injuries and develops standards for the health and safety of workers.

National Institute for Occupational Safety and Health (NIOSH): An office of the U.S. Department of Health and Human Services that conducts research and educational programs dealing with employee safety.

The Life You Save Could Be Your Own

6

ACCIDENTS ARE NOT like infectious diseases. They are not caused by germs or viruses, and they can't be eliminated by vaccinations or the right medicine. Accidents occur as a result of the interaction between the risks inherent in a given activity and human error. Although both risk and error are within the realm of human control, eliminating accidents is not as easy as it should be. Misinformation and resistance to change often keep people mired in unsafe behavior, and accidents go on happening.

Since early in human history, societies have tried to alter human behavior with rules, regulations, and educational programs aimed at coaxing reluctant citizens into safe behavior. Many of these programs have made a difference. Ultimately, however, we must take charge of our own safety.

SAFETY AND SOCIETY

Methods and measures to prevent accidental death and to minimize the consequences of accidents have existed for many years. The ancient Romans had traffic laws, including one forbidding bringing produce or goods into the cities during certain hours to prevent congestion and accidents. In early America riding horses too fast in the streets was outlawed to prevent injuries to pedestrians. Today accident prevention has become a science. Experts know that accidents are often caused by a number of human factors. Since accident causation is multifactored, so are the measures to attack the problem.

Did You Know That . . .

Primarily because of great-er safety consciousness and enforcement of laws against drunk driving, the U.S. death rate from all types of accidents fell more than 20 percent during the 1980s.

FIGURE 6.1
Driver Education

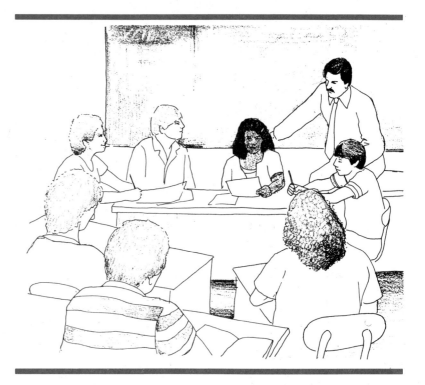

Driver education courses offered by schools and some employers emphasize defensive driving techniques, awareness of the rules of the road, and safety precautions such as the use of seatbelts and air bags.

Present-day experts have found that the most effective acci-dent prevention programs contain 3 components: education, engi-neering, and enforcement. This holds true for all areas where safety is a concern, including the road, the home, the workplace, and public recreation areas.

Education
Education is the first in the trio because most authorities agree that the best way to change risky behavior is through comprehen-sive educational programs that start in early childhood and continue throughout adult life.

Safety education begins during the preschool years when parents teach basic safety around the home and on the street. It

FIGURE 6.2
Learning Mouth-to-Mouth Resuscitation

A	B	C	D
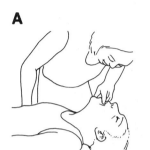	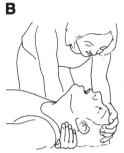	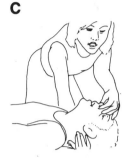	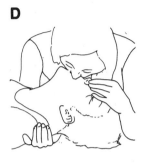

.**A** Use your fingers to wipe any obvious foreign matter from the victim's mouth.

B To open the airway, place one hand under the victim's neck and lift. Place the other hand on the victim's forehead and tilt the head backward.

C Pinch the victim's nostrils shut with the thumb and index finger to prevent air leaking out when lungs are inflated.

D Inhale deeply and seal your mouth tightly around the victim's mouth and blow into the mouth—full breaths for adults, shallow breaths for children, puffs of breaths for infants. Watch the victim's chest rise, listen for exhalation, and watch the chest fall. Repeat the blowing cycle.

When accidents do occur, prompt emergency care can save lives. Courses in first aid, lifesaving, and CPR (cardiopulmonary resuscitation) are offered locally through the American Red Cross, the YWCAs and YMCAs, and other local or national organizations.

continues in most elementary schoolrooms and in driver education classes in high school. In the adult world, most businesses provide safety training for new employees as well as ongoing programs for all workers. Managers of large companies have found that safety education is an effective way to cut their losses.

The challenge of safety education will be greater in the future than it has been in the past. Better safety-education curricula must be developed that will begin at preschool and continue throughout adult life.

Engineering

Safety engineering has developed into a broad field, ranging from automotive engineering to the design of safe toys and bicycles.

Safety engineering encompasses design, construction, plant layout, traffic flow, a safe environment, and much more. It is largely because of the efforts of safety-conscious engineers that companies are using sophisticated technology to design and develop safer automobiles, consumer products, and other goods.

Enforcement
There are thousands of new safety laws and regulations for homes, highways, workplaces, and recreation areas. Enforcement efforts aim to reinforce safe behavior patterns learned in educational programs and to act as a deterrent to unsafe behavior. These enforcement efforts involve more than traffic laws and regulations. Fire codes, building codes, occupational safety regulations, consumer products laws, and vehicle safety standards all play a part.

There is no single **panacea** that will effectively reduce accidents. The only solution is a comprehensive program based upon sound safety principles, effective **countermeasures**, and good management practices.

SCIENTIFIC APPROACHES TO THE STUDY OF ACCIDENTS

Before any program of education, engineering, and enforcement can be developed, safety experts have to know what behaviors contribute to accidents, where accidents happen, and who is most susceptible to them. To uncover this information, safety experts have developed various conceptual models.

The Epidemiological Approach
Epidemiology is the study of the occurrence of disease and disability. There are 2 basic types of epidemiology used in accident prevention work. The first is called **descriptive epidemiology**. Descriptive epidemiologists attempt to profile the frequency, consequences, and circumstances of the various types of accidents that occur within a given population over time. Using information obtained from sources such as police and hospital reports and public health records, descriptive epidemiologists gather and analyze statistics on accident rates, the resulting deaths and injuries, and the way in which these are distributed among various population groups. Descriptive epidemiologists are concerned with what happened and to whom.

Investigative epidemiology is concerned with the specifics

Panacea: A remedy for all ills; a cure-all.

Countermeasures: Actions an individual can take to prevent or minimize his or her chances of suffering an accident.

Epidemiology: The study of disease and injury as they affect groups of people, as opposed to individuals.

Descriptive epidemiology: The branch of epidemiology concerned with statistical measures of accident frequency and distribution.

Investigative epidemiology: The branch of epidemiology concerned with the specifics of accident causation. In this approach the cause is viewed as the interaction of a host, an agent, and the environment.

of accident causation. In this approach the cause is viewed as the interaction of a **host**, an **agent**, and the environment. Investigative epidemiologists seek to go beyond a description of what happened to determine why it happened. Their primary goal is to identify the specific factors that contribute to various types of accidents, and their findings are of particular interest to anyone interested in accident prevention.

The host refers to the person injured or killed in an accident. The agent of injury refers to the type of energy that caused the injury, such as mechanical, chemical, or thermal. Burns are an example of thermal energy, while a fall or a motor vehicle accident involves mechanical energy.

The third factor in the epidemiological model is the environment. Environmental hazards can be natural or artificial. Natural hazards include rain, snow, animals, floods, lightning, and dust. Artificial ones arise through disorderly situations, poor housekeeping, and poor storage of materials. Telephone poles and obstacles along the side of the roadway are examples of environmental traffic hazards.

The Haddon Matrix

William Haddon, Jr., has developed the **Haddon matrix** for analyzing the cause of accidents; it combines the epidemiological model with a series of phases. [1]

Phase 1: The pre-event phase includes all those factors that determine whether an accident will occur. Lack of education and skills, as well as the use of alcohol, are among the most significant factors present. Educating and training the host is the best type of accident prevention associated with this phase of the matrix.

Phase 2: The event phase occurs when forces of energy actually come into contact with the host. The countermeasures associated with this phase are those which moderate injury and prevent death. Seat belts in cars, football helmets for athletes, and leather clothing for motorcyclists are examples.

Phase 3: The post-event phase encompasses the measures, including emergency care, that are provided after the accident happens. Emergency signaling devices, such as fire and smoke detectors, are included here. So are the transportation and care of the sick and injured.

Systems Safety Analysis

Systems safety analysis, which was developed by the aerospace industry, is similar in some respects to the epidemiological ap-

Host: An individual who is injured or killed in an accident.

Agent: Something that produces an effect; a cause.

Haddon Matrix: An analytical tool invented by William Haddon for evaluating levels of accident risk and identifying potential and actual causes.

proach. When analyzing the safety of systems, the investigators examine the interaction of humans, machines, and the environment. They view an accident as part of a complete system in a logical order; they assume that the failure of one component will affect other components and possibly cause an accident.

ACCIDENT-PRONENESS

Statistics have revealed that some people have more accidents than others, and scientists have long been intrigued by this. Is it a coincidence? Are some people accident-prone? Or are all people prone to accidents in certain circumstances? Research into these questions has been carried out for many years, with controversial results.

According to some studies, much of the problem is because of statistical chance. For example, because taxi or truck drivers spend more time behind the wheel of a motor vehicle than the average citizen—professional drivers average 150,000 miles per year compared to 20,000 for nonprofessional motorists—they are statistically more likely to suffer traffic accidents.

Chance, however, does not explain the problem for all accident repeaters. Scientists have sought an explanation as to why some people suffer more accidents than others. The idea of **accident-proneness**, the subject of much scientific interest in the early 1900s, was largely rejected by experts in the 1950s. During the past 10 to 15 years some authorities have again been exploring the concept.

The most recent investigations of accident-proneness have led to 3 major theories:

The **multiaccident theory** assumes that certain accident repeaters are actually accident-prone individuals. Most studies have shown this concept to be invalid.

The **variable group theory** assumes that some individuals have specific characteristics that make them accident-prone. It also assumes that some of these traits come and go and fluctuate with time and with specific situations. Research has also failed to confirm this theory.

Revision of the above 2 concepts has led to the development of the **universal-susceptibility theory**, the one most widely accepted by professionals. This theory assumes that every individual has a different level of resistance or tolerance to accident-producing behavior. It also assumes that everyone is susceptible to accident-producing behavior, which varies from time to time

Accident-proneness: A tendency to be particularly susceptible to accidents; scientists debate whether some individuals are intrinsically more accident-prone than others.

Multi-accident theory: A theory of accident-proneness that assumes that people who suffer a large number of accidents are accident-prone people.

Variable group theory: A theory of accident proneness focusing upon the assumption that some individuals have certain characteristics that make them accident-prone.

Universal-susceptibility theory: A theory of accident proneness focusing upon the assumption that every individual has a different level of resistance or tolerance to accident-producing behavior.

(continued on p. 124)

Are You Accident Prone?

Some people just seem to be natural born klutzes. If there's a sharp-cornered piece of furniture within 50 feet, they're sure to walk into it. Show them a flight of stairs and they'll proceed to fall down it. Cutting knife in the vicinity? Somehow they'll manage to slice a finger. And, after each of these mishaps, they shake their heads and wonder why everything happens to them.

The fact is, most psychologists say, the things that happen to an accident-prone person aren't entirely accidental: Many of the things we call accidents are actually ways of expressing feelings that, for one reason or another, we can't deal with more directly. "Unconscious factors create a situation where we're vulnerable," says Bernice Rosenberg, M.S.W., a clinical social worker who practices in Peoria, IL. "We don't deliberately set out to hurt ourselves."

One frequent cause of accidents, Rosenberg says, is the tendency in our culture to push ourselves, to get a lot done. "If you find yourself dropping things, getting burned, and so on, you're not paying attention to your tasks. Perhaps you've overloaded your circuits."

Severe emotional stress—anxiety, depression, exhaustion, grief over a death or another loss, for example—can also interfere with your concentration and coordination and make you vulnerable to mishaps. Sometimes, even a moderate stress level can bring on a spate of accidents. Rosenberg points out that you may be more vulnerable when you're very busy nurturing others and not attending to your own needs.

In some cases, accident proneness can be an unconscious means of punishing yourself for something you've done (or even just thought) that violates your ethical code. A friend told me she had gone shopping, tried on an expensive, frilly teddy and toyed with the idea of shoplifting it. "I knew I'd never actually do it," she said, "but just the idea made me nervous. Leaving my parking space, I backed out too fast and hit another car. I didn't damage it, but fixing my own car cost $200."

Her unconscious impulse, according to Nancy Marks, Psy.D., a Teaneck, NJ, psychologist in private practice, was "I have to pay for my sin" or "I have to punish myself before someone else does" (even if no one ever would punish us). Similarly, Dr. Marks says, an accident can relieve a deep sense of unworthiness: "By hurting yourself, you're unconsciously saying, 'I don't deserve the raise I just got or the terrific person who's come into my life.' "

Sometimes, it's someone else we want to punish, but can't either because we don't dare or because the person isn't accessible. So we have an accident or a series of them. "Such accidents say something about your feelings of self-worth," Dr. Marks says. "A person who really thinks well of herself doesn't hurt herself or make someone else feel bad. There's magical thinking involved here, too, the childlike idea that you can *make* another person feel a certain way."

Many accidents are a cry for attention, help or love. A person who can't directly say he or she wants to be taken care of may manage to render him or herself helpless through an accident. "The only way some people can admit that they hurt is by making their pain a physical reality and therefore legitimate in their own eyes," says Dr. Marks. "A suicide is the most extreme call for help, and some serious accidents are actually suicide attempts." It's important to be sensitive to a pattern of repeated accidents as possible indicators that someone may be under severe stress or deeply depressed.

Accident proneness can run in families, points out William Fried, Ph.D., associate director of psychiatry residency training at Maimonides Medical Center in Brooklyn, NY. "Children can learn from their parents that having accidents is the way to express feelings and needs. Many women in particular were taught not to be aggressive," he says. "The aggression then turned inward, and the resulting hurt or helplessness was rewarded subtly or openly."

Accidents can even be metaphors for certain

states of mind. One woman I know has tripped on a cement sidewalk and fallen on her face twice in the past year. She has also been depressed over a series of career and relationship failures, and before the first accident had commented, "Whatever I do, I fall flat on my face."

Could you be accident prone? If, after serious reflection, you can admit that you're having more accidents than is normal, it's likely that you are. But you do have some control in the matter. Admitting your problem is the first step toward solving it.

Look at the pattern of your accidents. What was going on in your life when they occurred? Were you angry at yourself? At someone else? Were you ignoring your own body's signals of fatigue? Did you have needs that weren't being met? Was there something that needed attention, like a decision about your work or a love relationship?

When you've identified some of the factors that may be making you vulnerable to accidents, try to figure out how they can be effectively dealt with. If you're angry with someone, for example, talk to the person about it, instead of letting anger build up to the point where you may hurt yourself. "Don't ignore the fact that people you're close to may be unconsciously playing into your accident proneness," Dr. Marks adds. "Maybe you have trouble expressing feelings directly. Perhaps the person you live with has trouble listening. You need to talk to him or her about helping you share feelings."

However, if you're having serious accidents or a lot of close calls, you may not be able to change the pattern by yourself, Dr. Fried says. "You probably have moments of impulsivity, in which the consequences of your actions are unclear to you. In these cases, you should seek professional help."

Source: Gail Kessler, *Mademoiselle* (October 1983), p. 38.

according to the situation and personality makeup. Fear, anger, drugs, alcohol, emotions, stress, and other factors are among the elements that contribute to accident-proneness. [2]

A variation on this theme has been proposed by researcher Frederick McGuire. McGuire divides accident-prone individuals into 2 types: Short Term (Type I) and Long Term (Type II). [3] **Type I accident-proneness** is a crisis or short-term reaction. After the crisis has passed, the individual may no longer manifest the high level of accident-producing behavior.

Type II accident-proneness evolves from long-term conditions of personality, physical environment, or psychological factors that contribute to accidents. Antisocial behavior, senility, and depression fall into this category.

Type I accident-proneness: Accident-producing behavior characterized by a short-term high susceptibility to accidents.

Type II accident-proneness: Accident-producing behavior characterized by a long-term, intrinsic susceptibility to accidents.

PREVENTION TECHNIQUES

Safety scientists have also developed strategies for selecting the best prevention techniques for a given type of accident.

The Haddon matrix discussed earlier can help identify and select useful countermeasures. It is important to note that

FIGURE 6.3
Accident Rates by Type of Vehicle, 1989

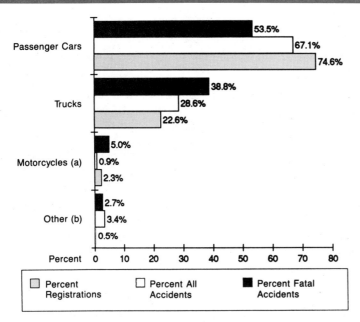

a) Includes motor scooters and motorbikes.
b) Includes school and commercial buses, taxicabs, farm equipment, ambulances, fire equipment, and special vehicles.
Source: Data from National Safety Council, *Accident Facts,* 1990, p. 64.

Did You Know That . . .

The term *accident-proneness* was coined by researchers in 1926, and the concept was supported by psychiatrists like Sigmund Freud and Karl Menninger.

Different types of vehicles have different accident rates. While passenger cars accounted for nearly 75 percent of all motor vehicle registration in 1989, they were involved in only 54 percent of all fatal accidents. Trucks, on the other hand, were involved in nearly 40 percent of all fatal accidents in that year even though they accounted for only a little over 20 percent of registrations.

Haddon's matrix is designed to reduce losses and injuries and not just prevent accidents.

Haddon has identified 10 types of countermeasures for reducing human and economic losses from all types of accidents: [4]

1. *Prevent the production of hazards.* Example: prevent production of explosives, all terrain vehicles, guns.

2. *Reduce the size of hazards.* Example: reduce the size of car engines, the speed of vehicles, the size of firecrackers.

3. *Prevent the release of hazards that already exist.* **Example:** ban dangerous toys, prevent the deployment of nuclear devices.

4. *Modify the amount of dangerous material a potential hazard can create.* **Example:** reduce the burning capacity of structural materials.

5. *Separate the hazard from the structure that is to be protected.* **Examples:** build pedestrian overpasses, place hazardous materials out of reach.

6. *Provide material barriers.* **Example:** use machine guards on power tools, build impact barriers on highways, wear safety glasses and motorcycle helmets.

7. *Make the hazard less dangerous.* **Example:** make toys less harmful, smooth surfaces, pad the interior of vehicles, soften play areas and structures.

8. *Make people and property more resistant to damage.* **Example:** implement driver education courses; implement tougher building codes for greater resistance to fire and disasters; build impact-resistant machinery and vehicles.

9. *Move quickly to detect an accident and prevent damage.* **Example:** install fire detection and sprinkler systems, provide emergency care.

10. *Stabilize, repair, and rehabilitate the injured person or structure.* **Example:** repair environmental damage.

How do we select the best countermeasure? There is no easy answer to this question. Some situations call for several measures, others may not require any. In his book, *Essentials of Safety,* the scientist and psychologist A. L. Thygerson lists the following as possible criteria for determining countermeasures:

1. Give priority to countermeasures that will best reduce loss rather than using unrealistic prevention techniques. For example, using a net in case an acrobat falls is more productive than simply telling him or her not to fall. Putting shoes on children is more productive than telling them not to stub their toes.

2. Combine countermeasures; a single countermeasure rarely solves a problem.

3. Give priority to obtaining positive results quickly.

4. Consider economic factors. The often-heard statement, "It's worth it, if it saves just one life" is not true if, for the same amount of money, more lives can be saved.

5. Emphasize simplicity. The less people have to do to protect themselves, the more successful the countermeasures will be.

6. Use the countermeasures that work best for the individuals involved.

7. Consider social, cultural, and political forces in the design of countermeasures.

8. Base the choice of effectiveness on reducing injury and death, not necessarily on preventing the accident.

RISK AND SAFETY

Some people resist accident prevention measures because they believe such countermeasures make life less exciting. After all, risk is with us every day and is inherent in many human activities. Life without any risk at all would be rather monotonous.

Safety pioneer Albert Wurts Whitney has developed a philosophical stance that views safety as an enhancer of life's excitement and joy.

> The very most right thing about safety is that it leads to a more abundant life. Safety in reality is substitutional rather than negative. It removes a danger but only in order to make it possible to take on another. Life is intrinsically dangerous. Life is partly routine, to be sure, but more fundamentally it is an experience of the unknown and hence based on adventure. A life without adventure would be stale and unprofitable. Safety would have a poor place indeed if it eliminated adventure. It eliminates an adventure only to make place for another and better adventure and the new adventure is often more hazardous than the original one. The prime quality in safety, therefore, is not the removal of danger but an improvement in the quality of adventure. [5]

In fact, most risk takers are very safety conscious and emphasize safety in their everyday lives, not only for themselves but for their families and others as well. Safety does not mean eliminating risk taking. It means minimizing risk while at the same time maximizing the quality of life.

AN INDIVIDUAL PLAN OF ACTION

The following plan of action can help you take charge of your own safety on the road, at home, and wherever accidents may happen.

1. *Identify the hazards associated with your activities.* Example: Capsizing is the most common type of accident associated with boating; speeding is a factor in a high percentage of auto accidents; hypothermia can result from a combination of wetness and windchill in wilderness activity.

2. *Identify the hazards associated with your age group and gender.* Example: Male drivers are more likely to be involved in motorcycle accidents than females.

3. *Remove hazards and reduce risk whenever possible.* Example: Drive within the speed limit; dispose of poorly insulated electrical tools or appliances.

4. *Use safety devices when hazards cannot be removed.* Example: Install smoke alarms in your home; always wear seat belts when in a car.

5. *Receive proper instruction for all potentially risky activities.* Example: Do not drive a motorcycle until you've taken a certified riding course; read instruction manuals before using power tools.

6. *Know the limitations of your equipment.* Example: The top rungs of ladders are not safe for climbing; riding mowers can roll over on steep slopes; overloaded extension cords can cause fires.

7. *Use protective clothing and equipment.* Example: Wear goggles when using weed whips or when using power tools that produce chips or shavings; wear life jackets while boating; wear helmets when riding motorcycles.

8. *Understand the risks that accompany alcohol consumption.* Example: Any activity, from driving to swimming, becomes hazardous when alcohol is involved.

9. *Identify the activities that are risky for dependent family members who rely on your judgment to provide safety.* Example: Children are the most likely victims of poisoning, suffocation, and drowning around the home.

FIGURE 6.4
Safety Equipment for Home and Work

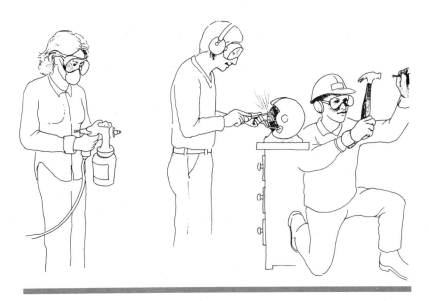

Air filter masks, eye protectors, ear protectors, heavy gloves, and hard hats are examples of safety gear that should be worn when using potentially dangerous chemicals or tools.

Learn to apply these basic principles of accident prevention and safe behavior to your activities. Understand risk taking and how it affects daily life, and understand the increased risk that goes along with the consumption of alcohol. Finally, be aware that making intelligent decisions regarding safety and risk is an essential part of every healthy and happy life. W

Glossary

A

Accident-proneness: A tendency to be particularly susceptible to accidents; scientists debate whether some individuals are intrinsically more accident-prone than others.

Acetylene: A colorless gas used chiefly as a fuel for high temperature torches used to cut or weld heavy metals.

Activated charcoal: A highly absorbent form of carbon that is used as an antidote for certain types of poisons.

Addicted: Psychologically or physiologically dependent on a chemical substance.

Agent: Something that produces an effect; a cause.

Anesthetic: A substance that produces a loss of sensation.

Apathy: A lack of feeling or emotion.

Artificial respiration: The rhythmic forcing of air in and out of the lungs of a person who is not breathing.

Asbestos: A naturally occurring fibrous mineral widely used for insulation and fireproofing; prolonged exposure to asbestos has been linked to lung cancer and other diseases of the lung.

B

Bilge: The lowest portion of the interior space enclosed within the hull of a boat or other such vessel.

Blood alcohol content (BAC): The percentage of alcohol found in the bloodstream; used to determine levels of intoxication.

Blood vessels: Any of the structures that transport blood throughout the body; the arteries, veins, and capillaries.

C

Carcinogen: Any substance known to cause cancer.

Cardiac arrest: A halt in the pumping action of the heart caused by cessation of its rhythmic muscular activity.

Carpal tunnel syndrome: A condition characterized by numbness, tingling, or pain in the hands resulting from nerve damage caused by the swelling of inflamed tendons and membranes in the wrist; it is associated with jobs that require repetitive motion.

Coma: A state of unconsciousness and unresponsiveness characterized by an inability to respond to outside stimuli.

Combustion: A chemical process characterized by the rapid oxidation of one or more combustible substances (fuel) accompanied by the generation of heat and light; the burning process.

Conduct: To transmit electricity; materials that have the ability to conduct electricity are known as conductors.

Contact dermatitis: A skin irritation resulting from exposure to nickel, detergents, medications, and a variety of other chemicals or substances.

Countermeasures: Actions an individual can take to prevent or minimize his or her chances of suffering an accident.

CPR: Cardiopulmonary resuscitation; an emergency procedure used to treat someone who is not breathing or whose heart has stopped beating by applying a combination of external cardiac massage and rescue breathing.

Creosote: A combustible, hard, black, lacquerlike deposit consisting of incompletely burned combustion byproducts that tends to accumulate on the interior of wood-burning stoves and flues; if allowed to build up to dangerous levels, it represents a serious fire hazard.

D

Descriptive epidemiology: The branch of epidemiology concerned with statistical measures of accident frequency and distribution.

Disability: Any bodily or mental impairment, particularly one that results in inability to pursue an occupation or activity.

Diversion programs: Programs designed to "divert" offenders from the normal criminal justice system into educational or therapeutic treatment.

Driving While Intoxicated (DWI): Operating a motor vehicle while under the influence of alcohol or other intoxicating drugs.

E

Electric current: A flow of charged electrons.

Electrocute: To kill by electric shock.

Environmental factors: Factors such as weather and road hazards external to the individuals, and any objects or devices immediately involved in an accident.

Epidemiology: The study of disease and injury as they affect groups of people, as opposed to individuals.

Epsom salts: A bitter, colorless salt consisting of hydrated magnesium sulfate that is used to induce vomiting when poisoning has occurred.

Ergonomic: Pertaining to the interaction of people and things.

Ether: A colorless liquid once widely used as a general anesthetic; full name, diethyl ether.

F

Fire extinguisher: A device designed to put out small-to-moderate-sized fires quickly.

Flammable: Capable of being easily ignited or set on fire.

Flash point: The lowest temperature at which a flammable liquid gives off a quantity of vapor sufficient to produce combustion if exposed to an open flame.

Frostbite: Damage to tissues caused by exposure to extremely cold conditions; symptoms include numbness and discoloration. It can lead to a serious infection, such as gangrene, if left untreated.

H

Haddon Matrix: An analytical tool invented by William Haddon for evaluating levels of accident risk and identifying potential and actual causes.

Halogenated hydrocarbons (Halon): Organically based chemicals formed by combining one or more hydrocarbons with one or more of the halogen elements—fluorine, chlorine, iodine, bromine, or astatine; such compounds are highly effective extinguishing agents, particularly for electrical (class C) fires.

Host: An individual who is injured or killed in an accident.

Hydrogen: An abundant gaseous nonmetallic element (symbol H) that is the lightest and simplest gas; it is highly flammable.

Hypothermia: A condition characterized by a subnormal body temperature, accompanied by drowsiness and significantly reduced respiratory and heart rates. Hypothermia is a medical emergency and can lead to coma and death if left untreated.

I

Ingest: To take in by swallowing; to eat.

Investigative epidemiology: The branch of epidemiology concerned with the specifics of accident causation. In this approach the cause is viewed as the interaction of a host, an agent, and the environment.

M

Multi-accident theory: A theory of accident-proneness that assumes that people who suffer a large number of accidents are accident-prone people.

Muzzle: The mouth or opening of the barrel of a gun.

N

National Institute for Occupational Safety and Health (NIOSH): An office of the U.S. Department of Health and Human Services that conducts research and educational programs dealing with employee safety.

O

Occupational illness: Any illness caused by conditions or hazards found in the workplace.

Occupational Safety and Health Administration (OSHA): An office of the U.S. Department of Labor that monitors job-related injuries and develops standards for the health and safety of workers.

P

Panacea: A remedy for all ills; a cure-all.

Peripheral vision: The ability to see objects and images on the outer fringes of the visual range.

Personal flotation device: A life belt, life preserver, or other device designed to help an individual keep afloat in the water.

Physiological: Related to or a part of the normal, biological functioning of the body.

Pica: A condition characterized by a craving for normally inedible substances; it is thought to be caused by a hormonal or nutritional deficiency.

Propane: A highly flammable gas primarily obtained from natural gas or refined from petroleum; used chiefly as a fuel.

Psychoactive: Having the potential to alter mood or behavior.

R

Raynaud's phenomenon: A blood vessel disorder characterized by the sudden contraction of the small arteries in the fingers and toes on exposure to cold resulting in their turning white, often accompanied by a feeling of numbness or tingling.

Rehabilitation centers: Facilities designed to help injured people by providing training and instruction in how to function with or recover from the effects of injury.

S

Sedative: A drug or agent that has calming effects on the nervous system.

Silicosis: A lung disease caused by the inhalation of silica dust; it is characterized by shortness of breath and decreased chest expansion and is most common among workers over 50; acute cases may develop after as little as 10 months of continuous exposure.

Smoke detector: A device that automatically sounds an alarm when exposed to smoke.

Sobriety: A state of soberness—as opposed to intoxication.

Spontaneous combustion: Combustion that occurs without the introduction of an external flame or heat source, usually as the result of the decomposition of organic materials or a similar chemical process.

Stimuli: Any external events or actions that prompt a response on the part of the individual who is exposed to them.

Stress: Any disruption, change, or adjustment in a person's mental, emotional, or physical well-being caused by an external stimulus, either physical or psychological.

Suffocation: A lack of oxygen caused by obstruction of the passageways that carry air into the lungs.

Survival floating: A technique designed to help swimmers and non-swimmers alike survive in the water for extended periods of time. Developed during World War II for downed pilots, it minimizes the effort needed to breathe while floating in the water by taking advantage of the body's natural buoyancy.

Syrup of ipecac: A liquid medication derived from the ipecac plant; used to induce vomiting when a poisoning has occurred; also known as ipecacuanha.

T

Toxic substances: Substances that are harmful or poisonous.

Type I accident-proneness: Accident-producing behavior characterized by a short-term high susceptibility to accidents.

Type II accident-proneness: Accident-producing behavior characterized by a long-term, intrinsic susceptibility to accidents.

U

Universal-susceptibility theory: A theory of accident proneness focusing upon the assumption that every individual has a different level of resistance or tolerance to accident-producing behavior.

V

Valium: Trademark name for a commonly prescribed brand of diazepam; a mild, psychologically addictive tranquilizer used to relieve anxiety.

Vaporize: To change from a liquid or a solid to a gas.

Variable group theory: A theory of accident proneness focusing upon the assumption that some individuals have certain characteristics that make them accident-prone.

Vegetative: A state in which one is unable to respond to external stimuli.

Notes

CHAPTER 1

1. *Accident Facts* (Chicago: National Safety Council, 1990), p. 2.
2. W. Haddon, "Advances in the Epidemiology of Injuries as a Basis for Public Policy," *Public Health Reports*, 95, 411–421.
3. *Accident Facts* (Chicago: National Safety Council, 1988), p. 56.
4. F. L. McGuire, "A Topology of Accident Proneness," *Behavioral Research in Highway Safety I* (Autumn 1980), 32.

CHAPTER 2

1. *Accident Facts,* 1990, pp. 6–7.
2. *Accident Facts,* 1990, p. 56.
3. *Accident Facts,* 1988, p. 25.
4. *Accident Facts,* 1988, p. 13.
5. Michigan AAA (private interview).
6. *Accident Facts,* 1990, p. 51.
7. *Accident Facts,* 1990, p. 64.
8. H. H. Hurt, "Causes of Highway Accidents," Traffic Safety Center of the University of Southern California.
9. Hurt.
10. Hurt.
11. *Accident Facts,* 1990, p. 52.
12. *Accident Facts,* 1988, p. 38.

CHAPTER 3

1. *Accident Facts,* 1990, p. 4.
2. *Accident Facts,* 1990, p. 97.
3. *Accident Facts,* 1990, p. 4.
4. *Accident Facts,* 1990, p. 95.

CHAPTER 4

1. *ATV Rider's Handbook* (Costa Mesa, CA: Specialty Vehicle Institute of America, 1987).
2. *NRA Hunter Safety Handbook* (Washington, DC: National Rifle Association, 1984).
3. *The Hunter Safety Handbook* (Seattle: Outdoor Empire Publishing, 1988).

CHAPTER 5

1. Michael Karter, "Fire Loss in the United States in 1988," *Fire Journal* 83 (1989): 5:24–32.
2. Percy Bugbee, *Principles of Fire Protection* (Boston: National Fire Protection Association, 1978).
3. "Avoiding Chimney Fires," *Consumer's Research,* October 1986, 28.
4. *Fire Protection Handbook,* 16th ed. (Boston: National Fire Protection Association, 1986), 20-4, 20-5.

CHAPTER 6

1. W. Haddon, Jr., "A Logical Framework for Categorizing Highway Safety Phenomena and Activity," *The Journal of Trauma* (Fall 1972): 12.
2. F. L. McGuire, p. 32.
3. W. Haddon, p. 420.
4. A. L. Thygerson, *Essentials of Safety* (Englewood Cliffs, NJ: Prentice-Hall, 1986), 46.
5. H. J. Stack, *Contributions of Albert Wurts Whitney* (New York: New York University Center for Safety Education, 1958), 41–56.

Resources

BOOKS

Brobeck, Stephen, and Anne C. Averyt. *The Product Safety Book: The Ultimate Consumer Guide to Product Hazards.* New York: E. P. Dutton, 1983.

Although almost a decade old, this book still contains important safety information on motor vehicles, household products, drugs, medical devices, foods, and toxic substances like motor oil and gasoline, and includes tips on safer products and their use. Arranged alphabetically by subject.

Hawkes, Nigel. *Safety in the Sky.* New York: Gloucester Press, an imprint of Franklin Watts, 1990.

This is intended as a book for young readers, grades four to seven, yet the author presents information about air traffic safety of interest to adults as well. The author discusses airline passenger safety and examines such topics as increased air traffic, aging aircraft, bad weather, poor cabin safety, terrorism, and difficulties with air traffic control. He also cites examples of famous crashes, provides maps of the world's most dangerous airports, and offers suggestions for improving air safety.

Jacobs, James B. *Drunk Driving: An American Dilemma.* Chicago: University of Chicago Press, 1989.

The author provides a clear and in-depth review and analysis of the drunk driving problem in America. Jacobs discusses the effects of alcohol abuse on traffic safety; examines the effectiveness, cost, and legal repercussions of many anti–drunk driving policies and programs; and offers solutions.

Knox, Jean Mcbee. *Drinking, Driving, and Drugs.* New York: Chelsea House, 1988.

This book is geared toward informing young people of the dangers of drug and alcohol use when driving. The author discusses how alcohol and psychoactive drugs impair coordination and judgment essential to safe driving. Knox also discusses the educational and legislative measures being taken to reduce the carnage caused by impaired drivers.

Stellman, Jeanne, and Mary Sue Henifin. *Office Work Can be Dangerous to Your Health.* New York: Pantheon, 1983.

Although dated, this book contains valuable safety information on indoor air pollution from photocopy machines and other common office machinery. The hidden effects of faulty office design are also addressed, such as inadequate ventilation, temperature control, and lighting. Information is provided on topics such as allergies, back pain, and factors that can cause sprained ankles or broken bones. The authors present detailed discussions of these problems and their solutions.

Viscusi, W. Kip, and Wesley A. Magat, with Joel Huber. *Learning About Risk: Consumer and Worker Responses to Hazard Information.* Cambridge, MA: Harvard University Press, 1987.

The authors present data from two studies that examine how risk influences behavior. The first study was designed to determine how consumers respond to hazard labeling. The second survey addresses the response of workers to hazard warnings and workers' attitudes toward their jobs when risks to safety and health become too high. The chapters cover a wide range of topics, from individual risk assessment to risk assessment in the workplace by employers and safety professionals.

PERIODICALS

Family Safety and Health is published quarterly by the National Safety Council and covers topics related to safety for children and adults. Articles include information on everything from first aid for children, to extinguishing small fires, to laughing your way to better health. A one-year subscription costs $7.98 for members and $9.98 for nonmembers. Write to Family Safety and Health, Sales Department, National Safety Council, 444 North Michigan Avenue, Chicago, IL 60611.

WOHRC News is published quarterly by the Women's Occupational Health Resource Center (WOHRC) and presents articles on issues concerning women's health and safety in the workplace. A one-year subscription costs $15. Write WOHRC, 117 Saint Johns Place, Brooklyn, NY 11217, or call (718) 230-8822.

HOTLINES

Auto Safety Hotline, (800) 424-9393. A service of the National Highway Traffic Safety Administration that provides information on driver and passenger protection and auto recalls. Also handles consumer complaints and makes referrals to other agencies. Operates 8 A.M. to 4 P.M., Monday through Friday.

Aviation Safety Institute (ASI), (800) 848-7386. Callers can access Fliteline service, which provides information on weather, delays, airport and runway conditions, and alternate flight routes for frequent flyers at any major airport. Information is also available on aviation safety and related subjects.

National Fire Protection Association (NFPA), (800) 344-3555. This hotline provides educational materials, information on fire code standards, and publications on fire protection, prevention, and suppression.

U.S. Consumer Product Safety Commission, (800) 638-CPSC. This service provides recorded information on household product safety, including hazards, defects, and possible injuries from cleaners and appliances. Accepts calls from people who report a product that might be hazardous or has caused injury, and provides literature upon request. Does not provide information on automobiles, foods, drugs, cosmetics, or industrial chemicals. Operates 24 hours a day, 7 days a week.

GOVERNMENT, CONSUMER, AND ADVOCACY GROUPS

AAA Foundation For Traffic Safety, 1730 M Street, NW, Suite 401, Washington, DC 20036, (202) 775-1456

This foundation works to prevent traffic-related accidents. Produces and distributes safety films, videos, and related materials for schools and senior citizens. Provides grants to universities, colleges, and research agencies for studies in traffic, truck, pedestrian, and bicycle safety, and drunk driving. Distributes materials directly to the American Automobile Association motor clubs, police departments, driving schools, and libraries. Publishes *Action Report,* semiannually.

American Driver and Traffic Safety Education Association (ADTSEA), 123 North Pitt Street, Suite 511, Alexandria, VA 22314, (703) 836-4748

Founded in 1956, this organization consists of teachers and supervisors interested in improving driver and traffic safety education in colleges and secondary and elementary schools. The association provides assistance to state departments of education, colleges and universities, state associations, and local school districts. The group publishes curriculum manuals, guidelines, pamphlets, public relations guides, and conference planning aids, and also produces audiovisual materials.

American Society of Safety Engineers (ASSE), 1800 East Oakton Street, Des Plaines, IL 60016, (312) 692-4121

Founded in 1911, the ASSE consists of professional safety engineers, safety directors, and others concerned with accident prevention and safety programs. The ASSE publishes *Professional Safety* monthly, which covers developments in the research and technology of accident prevention for professional safety specialists, including engineers, health professionals, and emergency planners.

Aviation Safety Institute (ASI), Box 304, Worthington, OH 43085, (614) 885-4242

Acts as an independent party not aligned with industry or government to promote and improve aviation safety. Operates an anonymous hazard reporting system, conducts safety education programs and seminars, maintains a computerized safety information system, performs safety audits and consulting services, and conducts aircraft accident investigations and research projects on topics such as pilot and crew fatigue. Publishes *Aviation Safety Institute Monitor,* monthly, to report on aviation safety, both civil and military. Also publishes research projects and other safety-related information.

Campus Safety Association (of the National Safety Council) (CSA), 444 North Michigan Avenue, Chicago, IL 60611, (312) 527-4800

Membership includes individuals whose activities are related to the safety of college or university employees and students. Publishes *Campus Safety Newsletter* bimonthly.

Center For Auto Safety (CAS), 2001 S Street, NW, Suite 410, Washington, DC 20009, (202) 328-7700
This independent nonprofit organization was founded by Ralph Nader and Consumers Union of the United States, and seeks to reduce the human and economic losses caused by automobiles and the automobile industry. The center monitors government agencies that regulate the automobile industry, supports safety standards, and participates in the rule-making procedures of the National Highway Traffic Safety Administration and the National Highway Administration. Collects and analyzes statistics on automobile safety. Maintains a library of 80,000 consumer complaint letters, coded by auto make, model, and defect. Publishes numerous newsletters.

Industrial Health Foundation (IHF), 34 Penn Circle, W., Pittsburgh, PA 15206, (412) 363-6600
Operates an analytical laboratory to study the prevention of industrial disease and the improvement of working conditions. Offers continuing education programs and provides extensive information on health control procedures, health hazards, and toxicity. Maintains a 1,300-volume library and biographical archives. Publishes *Industrial Hygiene Digest,* monthly, and technical papers for engineers and scientists in the field of industrial health.

Mothers Against Drunk Driving (MADD), 669 Airport Freeway, Suite 310, Hurst, TX 76053, (817) 268-6233
Over 1 million members belong to this group comprising 50 state and 400 local agencies. The organization encourages citizen participation in working toward reform of the drunk driving problem. Acts as the voice of victims of drunk driving crashes by speaking on their behalf to communities, businesses, and educational groups. Provides materials for use in medical facilities and health and driver education programs. MADD representatives serve on public, law enforcement, and legislative advisory boards and aid in establishing local, county, or state task forces. Provides victim assistance; supplies information for victims and their families on bereavement groups, the judicial system, and other assistance groups. Publishes the periodic *MADD National Newsletter,* the quarterly *MADD in Action,* and several brochures.

Motorcycle Safety Foundation (MSF), Two Jenner Street, Suite 150, Irvine, CA 92718, (714) 727-3227
The MSF is made up of leading motorcycle manufacturers in the United States, which seek to reduce motorcycle accidents and injuries through operator education, licensing improvement, public information, and research. The MSF maintains a 5,000-volume library of materials in the highway and traffic safety and education field. The foundation publishes *Safe Cycling* quarterly, which covers foundation activities and developments in the motorcycle safety field, as well as instructional, licensing, research and data, and consumer safety materials.

National Association Of Women Highway Safety Leaders (NAWHSL), 2826 Marshall Boulevard, Sullivan's Island, SC 29482, (803) 883-3419
Membership consists of women and representatives of women's organizations who work to reduce traffic crashes, injuries, and deaths by supporting and implementing the National Highway Safety Standards in communities and states. The aim is to develop more uniformity in traffic safety programs and regulations in all 50 states and Puerto Rico. Publishes an annual directory and several newsletters.

National Child Safety Council (NCSC), 4065 Page Avenue, P.O. Box 1368, Jackson, MI 49204, (517) 764-6070
A national organization dedicated to furthering the safety education of children by furnishing complete child safety education programs through local law enforcement agencies and schools.

National Commission Against Drunk Driving (NCADD), 1140 Connecticut Avenue, NW, Suite 804, Washington, DC 20036, (202) 452-0130
Consists of individuals and organizations concerned with promoting highway safety by reducing the incidence of drunk driving and resulting accidents. Holds public hearings and coordinates the implementation of recommendations by the Presidential Commission on Drunk Driving. Compiles statistics and produces a quarterly newsletter.

National Fire Protection Association (NFPA), Battery Park, Quincy, MA 02169, (617) 770-3000, and toll free (800) 344-3555
Membership consists of fire service, business and industry, health care, educational, and other institutions, and individuals in the fields

of insurance, government, architecture, and engineering. Develops, publishes, and disseminates standards, as prepared by over 100 technical committees, intended to minimize the possibility and effects of fire and explosion. Conducts fire safety education programs for the general public. Provides information on fire protection, prevention, and suppression. Sponsors National Fire Prevention Week each October. Maintains a 50,000-volume library of books, reports, periodicals, audiovisual materials, and microfiche, and publishes numerous journals and newsletters. Operates on a $33,000,000 annual budget.

National Safe Boating Council (NSBC), U.S. Coast Guard Headquarters, Commandant, (G-NAB-3), 2100 Second Street, SW, Washington, DC 20593, (202) 267-1060

Membership is made up of government agencies, volunteer organizations, and others interested in promoting recreational boating safety and in stimulating public education in boating safety habits and techniques. Major activity is observance of National Safe Boating Week every June. Compiles and distributes a promotion and publicity kit to help local organizations and field units of member organizations set up their program, secure promotional materials, and publicize the week. Compiles statistics. Conducts an annual boating education seminar in conjunction with the U.S. Coast Guard.

National Safe Kids Campaign (NSKC), 111 Michigan Avenue, NW, Washington, DC 20010-2970, (202) 939-4993

This coalition of national, state, and local organizations promotes a comprehensive childhood injury prevention campaign. The organization offers publications, pamphlets, and other materials to help increase the awareness of the seriousness of childhood injury, and provides programs to help local communities create a safer environment for children.

National Safe Workplace Institute (NSWI), 122 South Michigan Avenue, Suite 1450, Chicago, IL 60603, (312) 939-0690

Seeks to provide research and education on issues related to occupational health and safety and to make workplace safety and health an ethical and moral priority. Monitors efforts of the public and private sectors in improving workplace safety, and also monitors the U.S. Occupational Safety and Health Administra-

tion (OSHA). Operates litigation and legal resources programs and compiles statistics. Publishes *Information Sources/Workplace Safety and Health Issues,* semiannually, *Safety and Health Voice,* bimonthly, and national, regional, and state reports on occupational and health issues.

National Safety Council (NSC), 444 North Michigan Avenue, Chicago, IL 60611, (312) 527-4800

This voluntary, nongovernmental organization promotes accident reduction by providing a forum for the exchange of safety and health ideas, techniques, and experiences and the discussion of accident prevention methods. Maintains extensive library on safety-related subjects. Publishes numerous newsletters, technical publications, manuals, data sheets, handbooks, and booklets dealing with safety, and produces slide shows and films.

National Transportation Safety Association (NTSA), 836 NW 81 Way, Plantation, FL 33324, (305) 474-5938

Membership includes those concerned with accident survival in both air and marine travel. Seeks to encourage the development of equipment and refinement of techniques. Disseminates information to the public and Congress. Conducts research and development in survival and rescue equipment and compiles information on aviation and marine accident survival. Publishes *Gnat News,* quarterly.

National Water Safety Congress (NWSC), 77 Forsyth Street, SW, Atlanta, GA 30335, (404) 331-4834

Composed of individuals, business firms, state and federal agencies, and safety organizations that seek to instill safe attitudes and behavior in recreational users of the nation's waters and waterways. Promotes water safety through education programs, water safety demonstrations, and programs offered by civic and sportsmen's clubs. Compiles and disseminates water safety statistics. Publishes *Water Safety Journal,* quarterly, *Beach Safety Guidelines, Marine Safety Guidelines*, and other boating safety educational materials.

The Safety Society (TSS), 1900 Association Drive, Reston, VA 22091, (703) 476-3430

This organization is affiliated with the American Alliance for Health, Physical Education, Recreation, and Dance, and works to encourage quality safety education programs in schools and communities. TSS addresses issues of traffic safety education, emergency preparedness, health education for injury control, safety program management, and more. TSS encourages the development of safety concepts and behaviors among its members, and sponsors national conferences and safety programs. It publishes *Safety Forum* 3 times a year.

Specialty Vehicle Institute of America (SVIA), 3151 Airway Avenue, Building P-1, Costa Mesa, CA 92626, (714) 241-9256

This nonprofit association conducts ongoing research and field tests to study the safety of All Terrain Vehicles (ATVs), and produces pamphlets and brochures to encourage safe operation of ATVs. Supporting members include American Honda Motor Company, Inc., Yamaha Motor Corporation, U.S.A., U.S. Suzuki Motor Corporation, and Kawasaki Motors Corporation, U.S.A.

U.S. Consumer Product Safety Commission/Office of the Secretary, 5401 Westbard Avenue, Room 528, Bethesda, MD 20207, (301) 492-6800.

The Office of the Secretary is the primary contact within the safety commission for the individual consumer. This office answers questions, handles complaints, provides information on recalled products, and responds to requests for material. The commission produces numerous publications on all aspects of consumer product safety. Some of the topics covered include holiday decorations, playground equipment and toys, power tools, and kitchen products. The commission's library maintains a general collection of publications and periodicals on product safety, product lia-

bility, and consumer affairs. This is the organization with the legal authority to recall consumer products.

Tobacco Products Liability Project (TPLP), 400 Huntington Avenue, Northeastern University School of Law, Boston, MA 02115, (617) 437-2026

An autonomous project of the Clean Indoor Air Educational Foundation composed of doctors, lawyers, public health officials, and academics. Encourages liability suits against the tobacco industry in order to compensate victims of tobacco-related diseases and injuries such as cancer and burns, discourage smoking, and publicize the effects of smoking on health. Acts as an information clearinghouse. Publishes *Tobacco on Trial*, 10 times a year, which covers product liability cases against tobacco companies.

Women's Occupational Health Resource Center (WOHRC), 117 Saint Johns Place, Brooklyn, NY 11217, (718) 230-8822

The center functions as a clearinghouse for women's occupational health and safety issues. The goal is to increase awareness of the health and safety hazards women face in the workplace, and to raise management awareness of the need for improved workplace and equipment design. WOHRC advises manufacturers on design standards of safety equipment. Offers technical assistance in setting up programs designed to develop occupational health awareness. Publishes a quarterly newsletter, *WOHRC News,* in addition to fact sheets and bibliographies.

Index

Boldface page numbers refer to the pages in which the terms are defined.